the
heart of
garlic

Allicin's effective natural healing properties

An A-Z of conditions
and
suggested treatments

By Peter Josling, B.Sc. Hons.

Published by Natural Health Holdings Ltd in 2003

Printed in United Kingdom by Woolnough Bookbinding Ltd

Important Notice:
This book is intended as a reference volume only, not as a medical manual. The information given here is designed to help you make informed decisions about your health. Every effort has been made to ensure that the information contained in this book is complete and accurate. However, neither the author nor the publisher are engaged in providing medical advice to the individual reader. The suggestions in this book are not intended as a substitute for any treatment that may have been prescribed by your physician. All matters regarding health require medical supervision. If you suspect that you have a medical problem, we strongly advise you to seek professional medical help.

While the author has made every attempt to ensure that the information presented is accurate up to the time of publication, ongoing research may lead to changes in some of the concepts in this book. Neither the author nor the publisher shall be liable or responsible for any loss, injury, or damage allegedly arising from any information or suggestion in this book.

ISBN 1-9546507-0-0

Contents...

Chapter 5:   More serious conditions where allicin has been shown to be helpful

Part 3:   The Future

Part 4:   Little known facts and tips about garlic

Foreword...

t hroughout history it has been recognised that garlic has the potential to assist the immune system in a number of ways beneficial to our health, including the stimulation of immune cells, the killing of pathogens and the detoxification of carcinogens. But until recently the question has remained, how could we harness the special powers that the herb has long been suspected of possessing?

- Its use in cooking is widely thought to be health giving, and indeed it probably is to some extent, but mostly due to the range of minerals and vitamins that it contains.

- Garlic can of course be eaten raw, although most people find its pungent taste and lingering odour on the breath unacceptable. But even if we could munch our way through bunches of cloves the benefit would still be far less, than what we know to be possible.

- Many people select a garlic supplement from the wide range that is available. But as we'll see later, in only a very few cases are they likely to find a product which provides even minor benefit. What's for sure is that they won't gain the true benefit that is possible.

This seems a little strange. If garlic is so special, how is it that in all the three cases it appears to fall short of delivering its full potential? The answer is that the key active constituent, allicin, is a highly elusive and short-lived substance.

In this book you'll discover how garlic produces allicin, a sulphur-based compound with exceptional antibiotic properties, for its own highly-specialised purpose and how the compound quickly breaks down.

> "Only recently has it been possible to produce
> stabilised allicin on a commercial scale"

Only recently, decades after allicin was first identified in the laboratory, has it been possible to produce a stabilised form on a commercial scale. A team of chemists and chemical process engineers have pioneered and patented the unique process of water-based extraction and spray drying that made this possible.

This milestone achievement has finally made it possible for researchers to explore allicin's potential more fully and more freely, to confirm the most incredible spectrum of activity not only against a host of common ailments, but also against today's most pressing problems – resistant bacteria, virus and fungal infections.

You'll also read how such microorganisms could even yet prove to be the scourge of modern man, how diseases that mankind thought had been eradicated with the widespread use of antibiotic drugs are regaining footholds, and how important allicin is expected to become in the future.

"The availability of stable allicin means that the full benefits of garlic are available to the public"

Most importantly, the availability of stable allicin, produced in powder, liquid and cream form, means that at last the full benefits of garlic are available to the public. Later in the book you can read how allicin is active against an astonishingly wide spectrum of common and less-common conditions and how you can use it to fight and guard against these.

Do please remember that before following any of the suggested uses for allicin in this book, you are asked to give consideration to any health problems you may have and refer to a general practitioner or physician for advice.

"Allicin is nature's antibiotic, antifungal and antiviral"

Allicin is nature's antibiotic, antifungal and antiviral. I believe it has the potential to change the course of history. Provided people can get hold of it in whatever form is best for them, allicin has the capability to improve and even save lives.

I will give you a guarantee: Even if you are relatively fit and healthy, with no other complicating diseases, you *will* notice a difference when you start taking allicin. Within three weeks you will feel different, you may be detoxing your system and you will experience an improvement in your general health, wellbeing and resistance to disease.

Peter Josling, Director – The Garlic Centre

Part One
Chapter One...

A history of garlic – the source of allicin

To appreciate the importance of allicin it is first useful to appreciate the historical significance of garlic. Of all the plants used in cooking and natural medicine, it must be the best known and most widely used. This is not surprising given that its reputation as an "all-healing" herb has been solidly established over thousands of years.

"Garlic has established a reputation as an all-healing herb"

The use of garlic, the plant that is the source of the versatile ingredient and valuable restorative medicine, dates from Egyptian times. It was also popular with the Babylonians and the Hebrews. The great pyramid at Giza in Egypt bears an inscription indicating how much garlic and onion was consumed by the workers who built the pyramids. Indeed, it is reported that garlic was the cause of the first known industrial strike, caused when the ruling Egyptians stopped the daily ration of garlic given to the construction teams to ward off disease and build their strength. The men immediately downed tools and refused to continue their labours until the rations were restored! The Egyptians often left clay models of garlic in ordinary graves. However its powers seem to have been acknowledged at all levels of society for, during Howard Carter's 1922 excavations, six carefully-positioned bulbs were found in Tutankhamen's tomb – probably to ward off evil spirits.

Clearly the Egyptians were familiar with the power of garlic. According to records they were renowned for growing large tonnages of grain from which enormous amounts of bread were baked – the staple part of an average diet in those days. Unfortunately, this could often lead to problems with tooth decay. Milled flour often contained grains of silica from the sandstone mill wheels and this frequently led to premature wear of the enamel and tooth decay. The only remedy was to use the pungent qualities of garlic, as it was ground to a paste, and applied straight to the aching tooth! This rather hot climate was also infested with mosquitoes and other biting insects, many of which would carry malaria and other infectious diseases. Once again it was garlic that came to the rescue - as an effective insect repellent.

> ## F A C T
>
> Garlic has been established as a medicine for thousands of years and was well recognised by the Egyptians, Babylonians, Greek, Chinese, Vikings, Indians and Romans.

As time moved on, the uses of garlic in medicine flourished and many great physicians and philosophers made reference to its benefits. Hippocrates, Homer, Aristotle, Pliny, Galen, Virgil and Muhammad all believed garlic to have many useful properties. The Greek and Roman armies were, like the Egyptian workers, fed garlic to build strength, and the first Olympian athletes consumed vast quantities before competitions to build stamina and keep themselves free from illness. It was thought to be food fit for a god or goddess, and was placed ceremoniously on piles of stones at crossroads for the Greek goddess Hecate.

Ever since, garlic has been used by the dominant cultures around the world. Nowhere more so than in China, where garlic has always been used in both cooking and medicine. The Chinese call garlic "suan". The fact that this is written as a single sign in such an ancient language indicates a very early cultural recognition. Traditionally, the Chinese used garlic as an aid to long life as it was known both as a "healing" and a "heating" herb which helped the circulation and was believed to be beneficial in cases of tumours, tuberculosis, coughs, colds, infections and wound healing.

"Chinese believed garlic to be beneficial in the cases of tumors, infections and wound healing"

The Romans introduced garlic to Britain and it was later to be grown in monastery gardens. By the Middle Ages, garlic was well established although not necessarily loved by all! It was at about this time that legends emerged about its magical properties and its renowned ability to ward off evil sprits, in particular vampires!

The long pointed leaves are thought to have given rise to the name "gar", meaning spear or lance in Old English and "leac" meaning leek or potherb or vegetable.

BOTANICAL BACKGROUND

The natural origins of garlic lie in the steppes of Central Asia, where the plant grows wild. Other wild varieties grow around the world, usually in wooded areas. A member of the lily family (*Liliaceae*) garlic's botanical name is *Allium Sativum* (the cultivated variety). Other close members of the family include the onion (*Allium Cepa*), chives (*Allium schoenoprasum*), the leek (*Allium porrum*) and the shallot (*Allium ascolonium*). More distantly related are the autumn crocus, bluebell, aloe vera and lily of the valley. Of all the alliums, garlic is the most potent and the best known for its culinary benefits and its numerous medical uses.

Also commonly grown in Elizabethan country gardens during the 16th century, garlic became known as peasant's food. In those days the odour was considered offensive and was not greatly beloved of the middle and upper classes.

At about this time garlic acquired the country name of Poor Man's Treacle, which came from a Greek word for "antidote", which in Latin was *theiracus*. It was also commonly known as Devil's Posy and Witch Poison, doubtless due to its reputation for fighting off evil. Another name that became synonymous with garlic was "camphor of the poor", after its strong odour.

> "In the Second World War garlic was used extensively
> for its antibiotic qualities"

Much more recently two world wars saw attitudes move greatly in garlic's favour. During the First World War, the British Government offered farmers throughout the UK a shilling a pound to grow the plant. This was because its medicinal properties were being used to fight off dysentery and as an aid to healing and the prevention of bacterial infection in wounded soldiers. In the Second World War garlic was again used extensively for its antibiotic qualities.

F A C T

Aqueous garlic extracts contain plenty of beneficial sulphur that can unlock the full potential of plants and soil, when used as a bio-stimulant, allowing maximum plant feeding efficiency and this helps to prevent insect attack as well.

Part One
Chapter Two...

What is allicin and what are its medicinal benefits?

Garlic is remarkable for the number of compounds it contains, including seventeen amino acids, at least 33 sulphur compounds, eight minerals (germanium, calcium, copper, iron, potassium, magnesium, selenium and zinc) and the vitamins A, B_1 and C.

It also comprises fibre and water, but not a single trace of allicin, the wonder compound that this book is about. How can this be? It's a story of how a plant has evolved to protect itself from attack by microbes in the soil, and here's how it goes:

Alliin and Allinase. The Dynamic Duo.

In 1944 an Italian chemist, C. J. Cavallito, first isolated an unstable, odourous sulphur-containing compound with antibacterial properties from extracts of fresh garlic. He called the substance allicin (al-e-sin), after the generic name for the plant *Allium Sativum*.

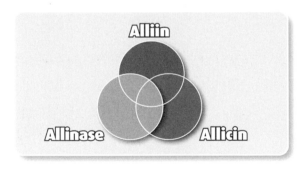

Four years later researchers Stoll and Seebeck, also working with garlic, discovered an odourless sulphur-containing compound called alliin (al-e-een). This they found to be converted by a second garlic constituent, an enzyme called allinase (al-i-naze), to form allicin.

The researchers made an additional remarkable discovery: When they studied cloves in cross section they found that alliin and allinase are stored in different compartments. In an undamaged clove they remain completely separate, but once its structure is ruptured – typically by cutting – the two substances come into contact and form allicin.

This transformation is extremely rapid, taking mere seconds. And even more intriguing is the instability of the allicin. It remains active only for a short period before degrading.

"The exceptional capacity of allicin to kill unwanted organisms"

There must be a reason for this. Nothing in nature exists without a reason. All the clues suggest that what garlic has evolved is a defence mechanism against attack from the soil-borne organisms. It has been found that invasion of growing garlic cloves by fungi and other soil pathogens causes the alliin and allinase to react, rapidly producing localised bursts of allicin which deactivates the invaders. This ability underlies the exceptional capacity of allicin to kill unwanted organisms, about which you will read more later.

There is a good reason why the highly reactive allicin molecules have such a short working life. If they didn't they would continue to react with surrounding proteins, including the allinase enzyme itself, and this would use-up the garlic's protection, which it might need later. This extremely efficient binary chemical mechanism ensures that the clove's defence is highly localised and short-lived – just sufficient to repel an attack. The remaining alliin and allinase are held in reserve to fight off any subsequent attacks.

While this is good for the well-being of a garlic crop, it poses distinct problems for anyone trying to extract and isolate the key active ingredient in a way that is beneficial. It was three decades after its initial discovery that allicin would be isolated in a stabilised form for the first time.

Mother and offspring
When allicin degrades, as many as 200 other sulphur compounds are formed. Many of these are transitory in nature, like allicin, while others endure.

One is a compound named ajoene (ah-ho-ene) after "ajo", the Spanish for garlic, which has been shown to possess antithrombotic, antimycotic (it kills fungal infections) and anti-fat depositing actions.

Others that have attracted scientific interest across a wide spectrum of disease conditions have only been used in experiments on animals, or on human cell models in the laboratory.

Thus allicin can be regarded as the "mother substance" from which all others flow. Raw garlic degrades into allicin to a greater or lesser extent and then many "sons and daughters" of allicin will form, some of which have beneficial effects on the body and some which do not.

So what is allicin?

In the opaque terminology of the biochemist allicin is described as *diallyl thiosulphinate, allyl sulphide* or even *S-(2-Propenyl) 2-propene-1-sulphinothioate*. What is important to recognise, is the most crucial and reactive part of the allicin molecule is the sulphur-sulphur bond coupled to an oxygen atom.

"Highly reactive configuration gives allicin its remarkable antibiotic properties, particularly the potential to assist the immune system"

Chemists know that this configuration is highly reactive, giving allicin its remarkable antibiotic properties and in particular the potential to assist the immune system in a number of important ways, including stimulating immune cells, killing pathogens and detoxifying carcinogens. Before the advent of pharmaceutical antibiotics, crushed garlic extracts were used to treat a wide range of infectious diseases including dysentery, typhoid, cholera, smallpox and tuberculosis. Then, in the 1930s, the first class of antibiotic drugs were invented, the sulphonamides. The reason they were so successful was the presence of the reactive sulphur group – exactly the same group that allicin contains.

How does allicin work?

Because allicin is so "keen" in biochemical terms to react with microorganisms, it is able to penetrate their cell walls. In doing so it is then able to upset their biochemical balance and impede their activity. At low concentrations of allicin, the degree of interference may not be lethal, but sufficient to block the microbe's virulence. At slightly higher concentrations the effect could prove lethal for the microorganism.

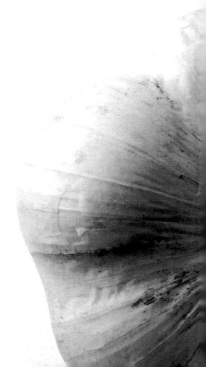

Part One
Chapter Three...

Do conventional garlic supplements work?

A quite bewildering array of garlic supplements are on offer, when you go into a health food shop or chemist, all apparently offering you allicin. However, in a review of garlic supplement brands carried out in March 2003, the independent consumer body ConsumerLabs.com found that the strength of these products, judged on each product's ability to generate allicin in a laboratory test, varies by as much as 1500 per cent. ConsumerLabs.com found that almost a quarter of non-aged products (aged garlic never produces any allicin) yielded less allicin than was generally considered therapeutic and then only in a laboratory and not in your body, which is an altogether different setting.

F A C T

The World consumption of garlic per year is approximately 1 clove for every living person!

In the UK alone more than two million packs of garlic supplements were purchased in 2002/2003 from chemists, supermarkets and mass merchandisers to treat elevated cholesterol, hypertension, and other common disorders. This makes garlic the most popular herbal product according to many sources. Yet NONE of those consumers are getting what they actually need from a garlic product – **that all-important heal-all, allicin**

Why? As we've seen allicin is created, when a garlic clove is ruptured, by the action of two constituents in a defence against attacking soil organisms. But just as allicin is produced in a matter of seconds, its potency dies away with the same rapidity. In its natural, unstabilised, form, it rapidly degrades and is simply not available as an active substance for humans to benefit from. In short, without allicin in its stabilised form, these supplements have little, and mostly no, allicin potential.

Consider the ConsumerLabs.com study in a little more detail. Thirteen non-aged garlic products and one aged product were purchased and tested. The amount of allicin produced by the non-aged garlic products ranged by a factor of 15 fold in the laboratory dish, which bears no relation to the environment of the human body. There's clearly no consistency of quality. Ironically, a product with one of the lowest allicin yields per gram of garlic claimed to be "allicin rich." Several products produced nowhere near the amount of allicin the manufacturer claimed.

"It is impossible for a consumer to know for sure how strong a garlic product is, without testing it," said Tod Cooperman MD, President of ConsumerLabs.com. "Few products clearly state their allicin yield and, when they do, they are not always accurate."

The important word in these statements is "yield". This is purely a theoretical amount and in the human body this just does not happen. The reason why, is that our gastric acids deactivate allinase, the allicin producing enzyme. It is estimated by garlic experts such as, Dr Larry Lawson and Professor Eric Block, that every time you swallow a typical garlic powder, 95 per cent of it will never become active, and you will get virtually nothing from it.

F A C T

Check exactly how much garlic is contained in your supplement, as some are virtually 'garlic free' and ask if the product has any published clinical evidence.

A recent paper published by the *Journal of Agricultural Food Science* by Lawson and Wang showed that most garlic supplements are standardised on allicin potential and are enteric-coated to prevent the action of gastric acid. To determine whether these products release the claimed amount of allicin under simulated gastrointestinal conditions (that is the conditions found in your gut), a standard method for drug release was applied to all 24 known brands of enteric-coated tablets. While all brands employed effective coatings and met their claims for allicin potential when crushed and suspended in water, 83 per cent of them released less than 15 per cent of their potential dissolution allicin release. Only when tablets had high alliinase activity and disintegrated rapidly did they show high allicin release.

Crucially the researchers concluded that garlic powder supplements should no longer be standardised on allicin potential, but rather on dissolution allicin release.

Further evidence was published in the same journal by two researchers from The Department of Chemistry at the University of California who analysed a large number of commercially available garlic products and concluded that the amount of allicin available from these products, when analysed in gastric or intestinal fluid, was less than one part per million (ppm). This compares with the guaranteed 100 per cent yield of at least 300ppm allicin from the true "allicin containing" products that are now coming to market.

What all this boils down to is that there really is *no comparison* between the general body of *allicin-claiming* products and the *allicin-containing* products that are now being introduced to the market.

Some garlic powder tablet preparations do have the ability to generate tiny quantities of allicin, and therefore all beneficial sulphur compounds that come from allicin will also be present, but as we have seen, the actual amount of allicin that your body receives from these products is minute. This is why there is absolutely NO DATA published on these products to show any anti-microbial activity, and even recent studies on cardiovascular activity have failed to confirm the promise that early studies showed.

What about raw garlic?
Eating raw garlic, which itself varies quite widely in its relative yield of allicin, is hardly an option, given the social consequences and, more technically, the deactivating effect of stomach acid on the allinase. In any case scientists have found that the amount of allicin released from different garlics around the world can vary by as much as 10 times, and given that the best yield is about a 4 per cent allicin yield, you'd have to munch an awful lot!

Or garlic oil?
Results of independent analysis from the Camden Food and Drink Research Association and the prestigious Warren Springs Laboratory show that garlic oil does not provide allicin. This is because it is destroyed by the boiling process used in the oils' manufacture. However, it is fair to say that some oil-based products do contain potentially beneficial sulphur compounds due to high levels of concentration.

Comparison of Garlic products

Type of supplement	Fresh garlic source declared on pack	Process to manufacture supplement	Allicin potential	Published blinded antimicrobial clinical data
Garlic Oil	No	Steam distillation	No	No
Aged Garlic	No	Aged over 2 years	No	No
Garlic Macerates	No	Crushed and dried	Yes	No
Garlic powder	Sometimes	Cloves chopped and dried under pressure and controlled temperature	Yes (Protection against stomach acid needed)	No
Allicin powder extracts	No	Specialised patented extraction process produces allicin liquid which is then spray dried	The product **is** allicin	Yes

Types of garlic supplement found on Healthfood Stores, Chemists and Supermarket shelves

Oil or water?

The method of extracting active sulphur chemicals from garlic is particularly important. Extraction using an oil seals up the activity of the sulphur compounds so that they will not readily be available to the body. Consequently, any activity is severely diminished.

Water-based extracts (like real allicin) are MUCH more active. This is the main reason why we see such good results against bacterial infections from allicin and ALL the other active thiosulphinate substances that allicin breaks down into. Products of water-based extraction methods are able to kill bacteria even when they are diluted 20-30 times more than oil-based extracts.

So if you want to produce an extract from fresh garlic that actually works microbiologically you have to use water as an extraction medium. The maximum amount of allicin is created. What's more the allicin is removed from the reaction so that it won't interfere with the continuing action of the allinase enzyme. Finally, to prove its effectiveness every batch of allicin that is produced is microbiologically tested against a multi-drug resistant strain of bacteria.

Clearly the mainstream garlic extracts are simply not in the same league as the allicin-containing products now on offer (see back of book for products that contain a guaranteed amount of actual allicin). With the advent of new technology one can now produce and stabilise allicin – the heart of garlic. This means that for the first time ever, anywhere in the world, we have the mother substance from fresh garlic ready to prevent and treat a wide range of common ailments. The next chapter details many of the conditions where allicin can really help you.

Part Two
Chapter Four...

An **A** to **Z** of ailments that allicin can be used to treat

The exercise of care in self-treatment

Although not a contra-indication, taking too much garlic can prevent blood clotting quickly and it would be sensible for people already on anticoagulants or those about to undergo surgery to advise their medical team before starting therapy with ANY garlic supplement.

Garlic can also cause reactions in people who are allergic, but this is usually mild and will disappear when you stop eating garlic.

After an operation is over it will usually be very sensible to start with allicin powder capsules as you will need to keep your blood thin and vigorously traveling around your circulatory system.

Because most people on the planet have already been exposed to garlic it is unlikely that anyone will be sensitive to any allicin formulation – if however this does occur then simply stop the treatment.

Garlic extracts have been used as medicines for thousands of years and the spectrum of conditions treated successfully is very wide indeed. The herb quickly became established as a cleanser of the body, a mild diuretic, a remover of poisons and a healer of wounds and sores. There is growing scientific evidence, including more than 1,500 clinical papers where activity has been proven, that allicin, the key garlic derivative, is the driving force behind a wide range of treatments and preventatives.

The following A to Z covers the commonest problems, which can concern us on a day-to-day basis with a suggested treatment regimen using allicin formulations.

ACNE

Medical definition

Acne vulgaris is a common inflammatory disorder of the sebaceous glands characterised by the presence of blackheads with papules, pustules and in more severe cases – cysts and scars.

Although the actual cause is still unknown many physicians believe acne is an infection. In particular *Staphylococcus, Streptococcus* and *Candida albicans* can infect tiny oil-secreting sebaceous glands found in large numbers on the face, upper back and chest. This leads to a worsening of clinical symptoms, and making treatment difficult. Allicin powder capsules and allicin liquid both routinely kill *Staphylococcus aureus, Streptococcus species* and *Candida albicans*. Their mild natural acidity is a big advantage as an acidic pH has been shown to be protective and guard against bacterial overgrowth. Thirdly, allicin liquid helps dry the skin quickly which in turn helps to shrink swollen lesions and assist in their removal. It also helps to pay attention to diet. Certain foods, especially sugar, caffeine, cocoa, refined vegetable oils and various preservatives, can aggravate the condition.

Treatment regimen

Take 2-4 capsules every day for at least 4 weeks. At the same time use a few drops of allicin liquid applied directly to each pimple and, if you can, add a few more drops to the soap or cleanser that you use each day. With regular use of allicin liquid and capsules significant results can be expected within 2 weeks. At this stage you can reduce the dose of capsules down to a maintenance dose of just one capsule each day. This is important to remember as it will help you develop a degree of protection against a further bacterial overgrowth.

ANIMAL BITES

Medical definition

Bites from pets are remarkably common, followed by bites from wild species and even humans. Any bite opens the victim up to any infectious organisms, which may be present.

A bite means that it is easy for microbes to get directly into the blood and surrounding tissue.

Because of this many physicians refuse to suture an animal bite since this would effectively seal the infection in. The result can be poor wound healing as well as the continued potential for infection. In this situation allicin liquid can kill a wide range of invasive organisms. Anyone prone to bites because of their surroundings or job can take allicin powder capsules to maintain a year-round background resistance to infection.

Treatment regimen

After you have washed the wound thoroughly squeeze in a generous supply of allicin liquid. This may sting a little but don't be afraid to persevere. Continue this 2-3 times a day for at least a week. The wound should begin to heal quickly. At the same time take 2-3 allicin powder capsules daily for a period of about 6 weeks to make sure you have sufficient allicin in your bloodstream to remove any pathogens that may be present.

Testimonial

I have used allicin liquid for treating a bite from a small dog as described above. It seemed to work very quickly and the pain was reduced in a few hours. I have continued to take the capsules and the wound has now healed. Mr DS from Bexhill-on-Sea

ARTHRITIS

Medical definition

Although arthritis literally means "joint inflammation," anyone who has one of its many forms or related conditions knows the condition often extends far beyond bones and cartilage. Examples are Sjögren's Syndrome, Psoriasis and Irritable Bowel Syndrome. By some estimates, as many as 70 per cent of people with Fibromyalgia have symptoms of Irritable Bowel Syndrome (IBS) - abdominal pain and bloating along with constipation or diarrhoea or alternating bouts of the two.

In the Middle Ages herbalists commonly recommended crushing up fresh garlic into a piece of muslin and winding it around an arthritic joint. This was to ease the pain and help reduce the swelling. Today we find that allicin combined with ginger is an ideal combination to take orally to help ease the misery of rheumatoid arthritis.

Ginger can help to relieve the pain associated with rheumatoid arthritis, due to its anti-inflammatory effects. It also has a warming effect on the body, which helps to relieve symptoms. The gingerols found in ginger attribute to its stimulating properties and heat promoting effects.

Treatment regimen
Take 2 allicin capsules with ginger 3 times a day either in addition to current medication or alone. The active ingredients will quickly get absorbed into the joints and help to improve mobility. This is a treatment that needs to be continued long-term.

ASTHMA

Medical definition
Widespread narrowing of the bronchial airways, which can change in severity over short periods of time. Symptoms include coughing, wheezing and shortness of breath. Caused by a wide range of allergens in the air, but aggravated by exertion, infection or stressful emotion.

The incidence of asthma is reaching almost epidemic levels. Not only are the death rates increasing but there appears to be no respite as we consistently challenge our body with poor diet, environmental toxins, excessive use of drugs and the fact that we are now constantly under threat from bacterial attack. It is also well known that simple infections like the common cold, coughs and sore throats can trigger an attack. Allicin can prevent and treat the common cold, coughs, sore throats and a wide range of bacterial, viral and fungal disease that can trigger classic asthma symptoms.

Treatment regimen
Take 1 to 4 allicin powder capsules every day and double this dose at times when you can predict an asthma attack coming on.

ATHLETE'S FOOT

Medical definition
This is a fungal infection of the skin, the scalp or the nails. Caused by the dermatophyte fungi – *Trichophyton* or *Epidermatophyton*. Its presence in animals is often a source of infection for Man.

The infection can be spread by direct contact or via infected materials, resulting in lesions that are often ring like and may cause intense itching. The commonest form is Athlete's Foot, which affects the skin between the toes. Another common type is ringworm of the scalp (*Tinea Capitis*) of which there is a severe form. Ringworm also affects the groin and thighs

(*Tinea Cruris*) also known as Dhobie, or Jock Itch and even the skin under a beard can become infected (*Tinea Barbae*). In research allicin in low concentration was effective against laboratory samples of *Trichophyton*, *Epidermatophyton*, and *Microsporum*. Allicin inhibits both germination and growth.

Treatment regimen

Simply apply one or two drops of allicin liquid between the toes and cover with cream. This should be done twice daily for between 4 to 6 weeks. Within a few hours the itchiness will subside and if it returns then another application should be made. For faster results use the liquid only as this is more concentrated. Once the cracking has begun to heal, patients should start on the capsules to act as a preventative against recurrent infections. As an alternative some people prefer to break open capsules and simply rub the powder over the affected area!

Testimonial

Mr KL from Birmingham, Alabama, started using the liquid as a treatment for Athletes Foot in February 2002 and continues to take allicin powder capsules each day. "The results are different to those of other treatments in that it does not dry out the skin but kills the infected tissue. Therefore, the incidence of cracking between the toes is virtually eliminated. The overall time scale is slightly slower than pharmaceutical drugs but it certainly keeps the complaint at bay. Interestingly it has not returned in over 9 months, which is very unusual as I often get recurrent infections."

BED SORES

Medical definition

Ulcerated areas of skin caused by irritation and constant pressure on a part of the body. Healing is prevented by a decreased blood supply. The formation of gangrene is possible and must be avoided.

This is an exciting area of research with allicin, since for many years we have known that garlic has two important functions with regard to healing wounds (see later section on wound healing). Not only can you expect to start healing faster but you will also prevent an infection from developing. Research is currently underway in this area.

> **Treatment regimen**
> Apply allicin liquid to the pressure bandage. Change frequently.

BLADDER INFECTIONS – Cystitis

Medical definition
An inflammation of the urinary bladder usually caused by *Escherichia coli*. It is usually accompanied by pain and burning on passing urine, with increased desire to pass water. A severe infection usually causes a persistent cramp like pain in the lower abdomen, together with fever.

Because allicin has such a wide spectrum of activity, and our results show a propensity towards drug resistant bacteria being the easiest to kill, allicin capsules will be worthwhile using against ANY microbial infection. Remarkably, allicin can kill *Escherichia coli* at a concentration of just 16 parts per million and we have even seen activity against a deadly strain known as *Escherichia coli 0157* at just 32 parts per million.

> **Treatment regimen**
> Take 3-6 allicin capsules every day for at least 4 weeks. Any vaginal irritation can be treated with allicin liquid 10 drops placed into plain yoghurt and inserted into the vagina.

BLOOD PRESSURE

Medical definition
The pressure of the blood against the walls of the arteries. Pressure is highest during systole, when the heart ventricles are contracting (systolic pressure), and lowest during diastole, when the ventricles are relaxing and refilling (diastolic pressure). The normal range of blood pressure varies, although with the typical western diet it tends to increase with age, but a young adult would be expected to have a blood pressure of 120/80 (systolic/diastolic).

High blood pressure is described as a "silent killer". It can creep up on you, without causing symptoms, to trigger a sudden heart attack or stroke. Even if your blood pressure is very high you may feel relatively well and symptom-free. Some people with high blood pressure may feel dizzy and develop a headache. People with hypertension will have high blood pressure reading even while resting. Factors that increase the risk of developing high blood pressure include increasing age, smoking cigarettes, obesity, excessive alcohol intake, a family history of heart disease, lack of exercise and high stress levels.

Medical experts reckon that reducing your diastolic blood pressure by as little as 5 units (millimeters of mercury) would decrease your risk of developing coronary heart disease by a massive 16 per cent. Allicin has been shown to significantly reduce both systolic and diastolic blood pressure. Recently the prestigious medical journal, *The Journal of Hypertension*, reported that garlic extracts with an available allicin yield of just 0.6 per cent could reduce systolic blood pressure by 10 per cent and diastolic blood pressure by 6 per cent. The journal went on to say that the potential blood pressure lowering effect of this natural plant medicine was of such significance *"that strokes may be reduced by 30 to 40 per cent and coronary heart disease by 20 to 25 per cent"*. We would expect to see both systolic and diastolic blood pressure lower by at least 10 per cent as a result of taking allicin products that can guarantee a genuine 100% yield of allicin.

Treatment regimen

While research is still in progress, testimonial statements from people who have experienced significant benefits while taking allicin suggest that you should take between 1 and 6 capsules a day depending on your current blood pressure reading. Allicin powder capsule products can be taken with any conventional blood pressure medication. There may even be a synergistic activity, which might allow you, under supervision of your physician, to reduce your drug intake.

Testimonial

Mr Steve B from High Wycombe writes:

Dear Peter, Just a note to let you know that I have been able to stop taking the beta blocker drug that was causing me so many problems and not really controlling my blood pressure. As you suggested I started taking 4 allicin capsules a day and monitoring my blood pressure reading. After 6 weeks I persuaded my GP to take me off the drug as I was having some personal problems with it! He took my blood pressure again 2 weeks later (whilst only taking the allicin) and to our combined delight my blood pressure was basically normal. I have kept taking the capsules you sent me but reduced the dose down to 2 per day and my last BP reading was still normal. Thank you so very much for your help.

BOILS

Medical definition
A boil or skin abscess is a localised infection deep in the skin. A boil generally starts as a reddened tender area. Over time, the area becomes firm and hard. Eventually the centre of the boil softens and becomes filled with white cells that the body sends to fight the infection. This collection of white cells is known as pus. Finally the pus 'forms a head' and drains out through the skin. Boils can occur anywhere in the body and affect people of all ages.

Boils may follow a bacterial infection, commonly an infection with bacteria called *Staphylococcus*.

> ### Treatment regimen
> When added to olive oil or apple cider vinegar, allicin liquid can be used to impregnate a lint dressing. This should be applied to the area affected and changed every day, and will quickly reduce inflammation and ease pain associated with boils and cysts.

CANDIDIASIS

Medical definition
A common yeast infection found in moist areas of the body. It is especially common in the vagina where it is known as thrush, but it is also found in the mouth and skin folds. On the skin the lesions are bright red with small satellite pustules. In the mouth it appears as white patches on the tongue or inside the cheeks. In the vagina it can produce intense itching and sometimes a thick white discharge. Candida infection can sometimes develop in people who are taking antibiotics or have a poorly functioning immune system. *Candida albicans* is often now resistant to a wide range of pharmaceutical antifungal agents.

The form we call thrush is associated with the overgrowth of the yeast *Candida albicans*. Around one in five women carries this yeast in low levels, but it can get out of control if anything happens to disrupt the body's defences. This could be caused by stress, low immunity, hormonal changes around your period, the contraceptive pill, pregnancy, diabetes or sex with an infected partner. Symptoms can include: intense itching of the vagina/vulva, constant tiredness, muscular aches and pains, mood swings, thick white discharge, digestive problems and, with oral thrush, white patches in the throat.

Treatment regimen

Start with at least 3-6 capsules every day, taken all in one go or throughout the day. This will need to be continued for approximately 1 month, depending on how deep-seated the yeast infection is. If you have a discharge then try adding a few drops of allicin liquid to plain yoghurt and apply this internally once or twice a day, again for about 1 month. This will have a cooling and soothing activity and should help to remove the itchiness that is so frustrating for many sufferers. Once progress has been made it is important to keep to a healthy diet, free from excessive sugar, and keep taking a daily dose of just 1 or 2 allicin powder capsules. This will help to prevent the infection from returning.

Testimonial

American Jane Jones, 35, lives in Kent, England and has struggled to manage recurring Candida infections since her teens.

The first time I got thrush I was only 15 and had no idea what it was. I had a white vaginal discharge and terrible itching – I thought it must be something to do with my periods, or that I'd catch something from a toilet seat. I kept it to myself for a few months until it became really bad. I finally broke down in tears and told my mum, who took me to a male gynaecologist. It was an awful experience, as he seemed to think I was sexually active – which I wasn't. It made me feel dirty. As I now know, although thrush can be transferred to a sexual partner, it's not necessarily caused by sex but by an overgrowth of the Candida fungus in the system.

After that first time, the thrush kept on coming back. My mum took me to a couple of female doctors who prescribed the same standard medication, which was Monostat 7 (I was living in America at the time). This was effective at first, but I think I became immune after a while, as I had to take it so often. The doctors also gave me the same advice: don't wear tight jeans, tights or synthetic underwear, avoid perfumed bathing products that can irritate the vagina and always use protection if you are sexually active. The treatments were very focused on the vagina and on curing the symptoms. Nobody ever mentioned dealing with Candida throughout the entire body.

A few years later many of the medications I was using became available over the counter so I didn't have to keep going to the doctor and it became easier to self-treat the condition. But the thrush still kept coming back, so I never felt free of it. I remember getting it badly when I was at university. The discomfort and itching were sometimes so severe I thought I'd go mad. I used to scratch myself until it hurt because the pain was better than the itching. I didn't confide in anyone about it. In a way I tried to pretend it wasn't there. I was shy around boys, and the boys didn't help my confidence. Whenever I had an outbreak I felt embarrassed and ashamed, even though there was nothing to be ashamed of. But psychologically it does get you down – you start to feel as if it's somehow your fault.

After university I went to live in London and then got married. During this time I started to feel generally tired and unwell. I was still having thrush all the time, but didn't relate the two – my doctor thought I might have glandular fever. I was reading up on the subject at the time and learnt that Candida overgrowth can have more widespread effects on the system, from bloating to chronic fatigue and digestive problems. I started to think that maybe I didn't simply have vaginal thrush; perhaps there was something going on in my whole body. I realised that when the Candida is really bad I don't just have thrush – I feel ill, tired and slow, like I can't think straight. One of the worst things is having no energy. I'm usually quite energetic, so feeling so tired for much of the time is very frustrating.

At this time of my life I was so unhappy that I let the Candida get me down. It was as though thrush was taking over my body, and I didn't feel like myself any more. I also thought the treatment I'd been having was simply addressing the symptoms of the problem, rather than the root causes, and that's why it kept coming back.

I decided to consult a nutritional therapist, who suggested I follow a strict anti-yeast diet. I was advised to avoid all fungi and products with fermented ingredients, such as bread, cheese and alcohol. At the same time I was, I was also taking a probiotic supplement, acidophilus, to help maintain my body's "good" bacteria and keep the Candida in check, and natural supplements such as garlic. My diet was something that I knew I could control and it was great to be able to do something practical, even though it was quite hard to stick to. I had to cut out all sugar, which feeds the fungi, so even seemingly "healthy" food such as fruit was out, as well as things you wouldn't think of, such as peanuts, as they contain a naturally occurring fungus.

I followed the diet for three months and it helped tremendously. I was symptom-free for about four years. Over that period, I gradually returned to eating normally – enjoying fruit, chocolate and sugary foods. I carried on taking acidophilus tablets regularly but I *almost forgot about the Candida. Then, about two years ago, I went through a stressful time, took two courses of antibiotics and within a couple of months, started to get thrush again. (I now know it can also be associated with stress, low immunity and using antibiotics, which can disrupt the balance of natural flora in the body.) I used Canesten cream and pessaries or Diflucan tablets and it cleared up. But it started to come back more regularly, and became so frequent I went to my GP to check my symptoms weren't connected to anything more serious.*

I was tested for diabetes and liver disease, which can both be characterised by recurrent thrush, but fortunately I didn't have either. I cut fruit and sugary foods from my diet again and started taking allicin powder capsules and vitamin C. I'd read about the curative anti-fungal properties of allicin in a book on garlic and found out that Candida albicans was one of the most sensitive species. I started on 6 capsules a day for about 4 weeks. At the same time I even tried aromatherapy, which is quite controversial as the treatment involves douching with essential oils and thrush sufferers are normally advised to avoid anything that may cause irritation. But I felt I had nothing to lose. Everything I've tried has had some kind of positive effect, though nothing has managed to keep Candida away for good until recently. It has now been 12 months since I started on allicin capsules and I now take just one a day – this seems to prevent the infection from returning, my life is now much more settled and I feel fit and healthy for the first time in years.

CANKER SORES

Medical definition
An open sore in the mouth, which appears as a painful white or yellow ulcer surrounded by a bright red area. A canker sore is benign (not harmful).

Canker sores are a common form of mouth ulcer. They usually appear on the inner surface of the cheeks and lips, tongue, soft palate and the base of the gums. They begin with a tingling or burning sensation, followed by a red spot or bump that ulcerates.

Canker sores are a sign of poor immunity and they can often develop as a reaction to toxic elements found in a variety of common foodstuffs that we eat. They can be triggered by emotional stress, dietary deficiencies and hormonal changes. They are often difficult to treat and tend to heal rather slowly. Most doctors now believe that they are caused by *Streptococcus bacteria*, which is capable of ulcerating mucous membranes. The cause can also be viral.

Treatment regimen

Dissolve 2 allicin powder capsules in a little water and then gargle for approximately 1 minute. Repeat this every hour for about 4 hours, then repeat once daily. You should immediately gain some pain relief and within 1 week your sore should have healed. Then continue to take 1 capsule daily for maintenance.

CELLULITIS

Medical definition

Cellulitis is defined as large-scale inflammation and infection of the connective tissue between adjacent tissues and organs. This is commonly due to bacterial infection by *Streptococci species* and occasionally by *Staphylococci species*.

It is important to stop the infection spreading to the bloodstream as this can lead to serious problems that could require hospitalisation.

Treatment regimen

If the infection is mild and manifests itself on the skin then apply a few drops of allicin liquid to each abrasion, twice daily. Supplement this treatment with at least 4 allicin powder capsules daily and continue this regimen for 14 days. If you have a long-term infection that has not been touched by successive courses of antibiotics then it is important to double the dose of allicin powder capsules and stay on this increased dose for at least 3 months. When there is a sign of any improvement then it would be possible to reduce the dose down to 1-2 capsules a day.

CHOLESTEROL

Medical definition

A fat-like material present in the blood and in most tissues. Cholesterol is an important constituent of cell membranes and the precursor to many steroid hormones and bile salts. Western dietary intake of cholesterol is approximately 500-1000mg per day.

Cholesterol is synthesised in the body from acetate, mainly in the liver and blood concentration should be between 100-300mg/dL. Elevated levels of cholesterol are associated with atheroma and need to be controlled.

POOR BLOOD CIRCULATION

Medical definition

There are many factors that lead to poor blood circulation, including atherosclerosis, hypertension, coronary artery disease, carotid artery disease, peripheral artery disease and heart disease. The results of these are: Angina pectoris (chest pain), limitation of movement, memory loss, stroke, cardiac arrhythmias, myocardial infarctions, congestive heart failure, valvular heart disease and cold hands and feet.

There is evidence that allicin may help to improve circulation in several ways. By making your blood less likely to clot, allicin can reduce blood platelet aggregation. This means that your blood will become slightly thinner and is less likely to form a clot since the platelets are prevented from sticking together. It has also been reported that allicin can reduce blood thickening. In one study, which looked at capillary blood flow in the nail folds of the hand, allicin was found to increase blood flow by 55 per cent. As soon as you take an allicin capsule your blood immediately thins and becomes more mobile. It will return to normal within about three hours once the active metabolites that allicin breaks down into have done their work and have been excreted.

Treatment regimen
Take 1 to 4 capsules every day, especially during the winter months.

COLD SORES

Medical definition

Inflammation of the skin or mucus membranes caused by herpes virus and is characterised by a collection of small blisters especially on the lips. *Herpes simplex* virus (HSV 1) causes the common cold sore and HSV-2 is responsible for genital herpes. Both types can cause either genital herpes or cold sores depending on the site of the initial infection. HSV blisters are contagious through skin-to-skin contact and are recurrent in many people.

Most people who are afflicted with recurrent cold sores know exactly when an attack is coming. They will get a tingle on the lips and if you take action fast enough with allicin liquid you can prevent that tingle from becoming a full-blown painful cold sore. Herpes infection arises as a result of some type of toxic insult, which could be stress, infectious illness, food allergies, drug or alcohol abuse, too much sunlight or cold exposure. A significant number of pharmaceutical drugs can also trigger a reaction including, aspirin, Motrin, Indocin, Clinoril and Cardizem. Procardia and cortisone are known to increase the invasive nature of herpes virus.

Treatment regimen
Apply just 1 drop of allicin liquid to the sore spot 2 or 3 times a day and this will prevent it from developing into a serious cold sore. At the same time take 2-4 capsules of allicin powder a day and continue this especially through periods where you might expect to suffer. This protocol should help to prevent the infection from flaring up again.

Testimonials
I have not had any cold sores on my lips since I have started the treatment. One on the tip of my nose and I think that was my husband's fault, as he had one on his lip. This is the longest time I have experienced being without sore lips, so a thank you very much for all your help.
Shena P, Portland, Oregon

I can always tell when a cold sore is coming as my lip begins to tingle and I know that if I don't take action immediately then in the next few days I will get a terribly ugly and painful cold sore. I was given some of your allicin liquid to try and I first applied just a couple of drops when I felt the tingle. To my amazement and delight the expected cold sore did not develop at all. I continued to apply the liquid for a few days and although it has a characteristic smell – this disappeared within minutes of application. Thank you very much for a simple, natural and effective treatment for my cold sores.
Agnes B, Rye, East Sussex, England

COLDS and INFLUENZA

Medical definition
Experts in colds and flu like Professor Ron Eccles, who runs The Common Cold Centre, will confirm that it is very difficult to determine the difference between a bad cold and a mild flu. Classic cold symptoms are headache, fever, malaise, muscle aches and pains, earache, sinus pain, cough, sneezing, runny nose, sore throat and a blocked nose. Influenza is a highly contagious viral infection that affects the respiratory system.

Flu viruses are transmitted by coughing and sneezing. Symptoms commence after an incubation period of 1-4 days and include headaches, fever, loss of appetite, weakness, sore throat, sneezing, runny nose and general aches and pains. They may continue for about a week but a few may go onto develop pneumonia either a primary influenzal viral pneumonia or a secondary bacterial pneumonia. The main bacterial organisms responsible for a secondary infection include *Streptococcus pneumonia*, *Haemophilus influenza* and *Staphylococcus aureus*. All of these bacteria are destroyed by allicin powder capsules.

Treatment regimen

For prevention studies have shown that just 1 capsule of allicin powder per day can prevent the common cold. If you are already suffering then double or triple the dose for a period of up to 7 days and this will relieve the symptoms to leave you feeling much better.

Testimonials

Mr CP from Rye in Sussex writes: "When I started a heavy cold and initially took 4 capsules per day for the duration of the cold. The first thing that struck me was that the runny nose cleared up much faster that it would have normally. I continued with 4 a day until the worst of the cold was over. I also noted that the usual aftermath of mucus (which usually hangs about because I smoke) was not as severe and cleared more quickly. From that date I reduced the intake to 1 cap per day until I ran out last week! Coincidentally or not the following day I came down with another heavy cold and unfortunately I did not take any capsules until the end of the week. I immediately took 4 capsules, and have continued until now which is a week from the start. I won't say my cold has cleared but it is much better. I can breathe clearly and the congestion is beginning to clear (loosen). As you know I was very congested on Friday last. The other thing, which occurs to me, is that I normally feel dreadful when I have a cold for at least 4-5 days, to the point where I do not feel like doing anything. This time I only felt that bad for two days, i.e. Wednesday and Thursday. However, on Friday and through the weekend my energy levels were good despite the fact that I was still heady from cold. The other side effect of taking allicin I have found is not one of a laxative but more of a regulariser despite the fact that my dietary habits have not changed. This may be coincidence I do not know. There can be little doubt that that allicin has beneficial effects as I am a firm believer that treatment from within is the best way to combat ailments and if the digestive system is working correctly then the body will do the rest. Incidentally, during this time I have only taken the occasional Paracetemol at night to combat headaches."

Mr CF from Sheerness, Kent, England writes

Dear Peter,

On taking allicin powder capsules for the first time I encountered several positive experiences, I started to realise a huge "clearing" of the airways, almost a slightly runny/mucusey cold. As this started to diminish I noticed, it seemed, I could draw large volumes of air through my nose or mouth, like I had not done for a good while, what I would call really clear breathing. My wife also commented that I seemed to snore less at this time.

I continued to take allicin powder capsules on a maintained dose of 1-2 capsules every other day depending on how I felt. During this period of approx 6 months I never contracted a cold and had good health despite being in the company of others who had colds. Then, after stopping the allicin powder capsules for approx 6 weeks, I contracted a really severe cold. Straight away I started allicin powder capsules again. Within 2 days there was a noticeable improvement. The allicin powder capsules seemed to be reducing the symptoms of the cold; I was certainly recovering quicker than a colleague at work. Then I ran out of allicin powder capsules. This proved to be a disaster, the cold returned with a vengeance. $1\frac{1}{2}$ days after running out, the cold was worse than ever. On restarting the allicin powder capsules the cold symptoms started to lessen, but it proved difficult to shake off, until I doubled the dose this was large enough to kill it off the second time. A cold like this would always go to my chest and result in a sore throat, but this time it hasn't. This is very unusual.

Dosage I took:

As an everyday supplement 1-2 capsules twice a day for 3 days (to start), then 1-2 capsules every other day as maintenance.

As a cold cure: 2 x 2 capsules every day (this may have needed to be more)

Mrs PMI also from Kent is a sufferer of multiple sclerosis. This means that she has a severely compromised immune system and in previous years has always been highly susceptible to infections. She writes:

Dear Sirs,

Having MS and having no effective immune system I am certain that taking allicin powder capsules over the past winter months has helped to protect me from colds and flu. I am pleased to inform you, therefore, that allicin powder capsules with 100 per cent allicin will be a definite part of my future daily intake.

Thank you so much,

Patricia

COUGH and upper respiratory tract infections

Medical definition

The upper part of the respiratory tract is responsible for warming, humidifying and purifying the air that comes into our body. It is therefore this area that is likely to become damaged by pollution or infected by bacteria or viruses. The mucus membranes that make up the upper respiratory tract, when under stimulation, secrete mucus, and it is this that leads to a stuffy nose, sinusitis, earache or a chronic cough.

An unrelenting cough is most annoying and yet in many cases the true cause is never discovered. We do know that it can be a deep-seated bacterial cause or, where it is caused by a cold it is usually a viral infection. Allicin is good for chest complaints, especially troublesome and persistent coughs, since it has a major antitussive activity. Unlike most over-the-counter medicines allicin powder capsules can destroy both bacterial and viral organisms with consummate ease. This can be achieved in several ways.

Treatment regimen

Put 10 drops of allicin liquid in a small cupful of warm milk and gargle for a few minutes. Do this every night for a few days. Then before retiring to bed take 6 allicin powder capsules and continue this until the cough begins to break up. Then reduce the dose down to 4 and then to 2 after a further week.

CRYPTOSPORIDIUM

Medical definition

A parasitic infection caused by a protozoan that comes from infected human and animal excrement, commonly found in soil and fresh water. In recent years this has become a much more widespread problem.

In 1993 approximately 400,000 Milwaukee residents were reported to have developed the infection from drinking contaminated water, and dozens died. Recent infections in Great Britain and Canada were also traced to contaminated water supplies and large populations were required to boil water for domestic use for several months. No effective drug medications or water sterilants are available and this parasite remains a cause for concern.

Treatment regimen

Treatment needs to be aggressive and prolonged to have a chance of destroying this parasite. A large dose of up to 10 allicin powder capsules a day should be taken all at once or spread throughout the day. It would also be sensible to take 10 drops of allicin liquid in fruit juice twice a day for the entire treatment period. Results will depend on each individual's response – but don't be afraid to persevere as the allicin can only do you good.

DANDRUFF

Medical definition

Visible scaling from the scalp is common and evident in at least 50 per cent of the population. Dandruff is caused by the yeast *Pityrosporum ovale*, and is often the precursor of seborrhoeic eczema of the scalp. This is usually accompanied by a degree of inflammation and greasy scaling.

Most people don't realize that dandruff is caused by a fungal infection and most proprietary shampoos and conditioners just do not contain any antifungal agents at all. Consequently very little impact is made, and yet a huge amount of money is spent on the latest cosmetic products, which promise success. Allicin liquid can be mixed with any shampoo or conditioner and just a few applications will get rid of dandruff very easily. Again it is necessary to adopt the "heal from within and heal from without" principle. This means that you must start taking allicin powder capsules at the same time, since we are trying to get rid of an infection and then prevent it from coming back.

Treatment regimen

Add 8 drops of allicin liquid to a normal measure of shampoo and massage as usual in the last wash. You can then use a conditioner if necessary. Repeat this every time you wash your hair for about 1 month. At the same time start taking just 1 capsule of allicin powder every day and continue this to help prevent the infection from returning.

DIABETES

Medical definition

There are two major types of diabetes: juvenile-onset and maturity-onset.

The symptoms of juvenile-onset diabetes come on very dramatically and rapidly because the beta cells in the pancreas are producing little or no insulin. Insulin shots are required to manage juvenile-onset diabetes.

The symptoms of mature-onset diabetes appear more gradually, and can be treated by diet and tablets alone. Occasionally insulin injections may be necessary. In mature-onset diabetes, the beta cells in the pancreas still produce insulin, but it is the insulin receptors that become less sensitive to the insulin. Hence mature-onset diabetics have to control their blood sugar levels too.

Diabetics are three times more likely to suffer from cardiovascular disease than a normal individual, are less able to fight off infections and will heal much more slowly than non-diabetics. Allicin powder capsules can offer a cascade of benefits to people suffering from diabetes.

Treatment regimen

To keep your circulation fit and healthy take two allicin powder capsules every day. Use the liquid, as detailed below, for treating minor wounds.

The author's own experience

As the author of this book I have a unique experience with the production and application of allicin. I am also a diabetic of some 32 years standing so anything I can do to reduce the risks detailed above has to be good for me. Consequently I take allicin capsules every day to help keep my blood pressure, cholesterol and circulation fit and healthy. Anyone who knows me will tell you that before the advent of allicin powder capsules, I used to take a popular garlic powder supplement and every year around October time I would get a real stinker of a cold. This would inevitably last at least 10 days as my immune system doesn't function as well as a non-diabetic and my blood sugar levels would go haywire. Since starting allicin powder capsules several years ago I have not had ANY colds despite now having 2 young children at school! I can only put this down to allicin.

Diabetics, myself included, also tend to heal very slowly. I still have a scar from a minor burn I sustained when I was a teenager and every time I cut myself it seems to take ages to heal properly. However, recently I have started putting allicin liquid onto plasters or bandages used to dress small cuts and grazes. A short time ago I got a nasty wood splinter in my thumbnail. I managed to remove it but immediately it started to swell up a little and became very painful. I immediately added just 3 drops of allicin liquid to a band-aid and dressed the wound. Literally within a few hours the pain and swelling had begun to reduce. The next day, I changed the dressing and within 3-4 days the wound had healed, the swelling had gone and it was not painful at all. Several days later, having stopped the treatment, my skin began to flake and peel away leaving a perfectly healed thumb – allicin really is great stuff for diabetics.

DIARRHOEA

Medical definition
Frequent bowel evacuation or the passage of abnormally soft or liquid faeces. This is often caused by intestinal infection especially by *Escherichia coli*. Severe or prolonged diarrhoea may lead to extreme loss of fluids, salt and nutrients.

I can personally guarantee that this works. As a person who sometimes gets a stomach upset that leads to terrible stomach pains followed by the classic "explosion", I have in the past relied on pharmaceutical preparations, which certainly do work. However, currently I much prefer to use allicin as it is safe, natural and very effective!

Treatment regimen
You can get rid of this type of problem very easily with allicin powder capsules. All you need to do is take a large dose - once and this will get rid of an upset stomach. Take 6 capsules in one go. This may have to be repeated six hours later.

EAR INFECTIONS

Medical definition
Middle ear infection, or Otitis media, is one of the commonest of childhood complaints and tends to occur whenever there is a blockage of the Eustachian tube at the lower end on account of catarrh or enlarged adenoids. If a cold or other respiratory infection occurs then it

will often progress upward into the middle ear and cause pain of a stabbing or throbbing nature. The secretions will become infected with *Staphylococci* or *Streptococci bacteria*.

Ear infections are particularly difficult to live with, especially for children, who tend to suffer more than adults. It can be impossible for your child to communicate the pain and discomfort they are suffering. As a caring parent you naturally want to get a quick resolution. A trip to the doctor will result in a prescription for an antibiotic drug which may work – but a cursory look at the medical databases shows that when children are aggressively treated with antibiotics they become 300 percent more likely to develop recurrent infections when compared to those who have no treatment at all. Overuse of antibiotics often causes another problem; since children are still developing an effective immune system, they can easily end up with a fungal infection.

Treatment regimen
Any condition that has a microbial cause can be treated with allicin. Children younger than 7 years can be given half a capsule a day. Children over 7 years, the normal adult dose of 1 capsule a day. Split the capsules open and place the powder in their food. You can also drizzle the liquid into the ear just 1 drop at a time for a period of up to 1 week.

ECZEMA

Medical definition
This is a common itchy skin disease characterised by reddening and vesicle formation, which may lead to weeping and crusting. Atopic eczema affects up to 20 per cent of the population and is associated with hay fever and asthma. It can affect young children in particular where the disease may last for several years and may lead on into adulthood.

Most people who suffer from eczema will have their own treatment routine to keep the disease at bay. It could involve a number of pharmaceutical agents including steroids plus emollients, or any of a number of herbal remedies. However most sufferers will also report that these treatments work for a while and then cease to be effective. One of the major reasons for this is that NONE of them (including pharmaceutical drugs) kill the bacterium found in 95 per cent of simple eczema cases – *Staphylococcus aureus*. This bug is frequently found all over the skin surface of eczema sufferers. This bacterium is clever and will selectively seek out a route into the human body (see MRSA section later) so an eczema patient is the ideal vehicle for *Staphylococcus aureus* to replicate on and infect. The bacterium's presence on the skin will cause a secondary infection, which leads to a worsening of clinical symptoms and also hinders the absorption of hydrocortisone. So it stands to reason that you must use an agent that can kill *Staphyloccocus aureus* and allow the underlying disease to heal. Allicin can do this easily. So far over 80 strains of this infectious, multi-drug resistant bacterium have been tested against allicin liquid, powder and cream formulations and have all been blown away!

Treatment regimen
Begin by starting a high dose course of allicin powder capsules. Take up to 6 a day. At the same time take a few drops of allicin liquid or cream and apply sparingly to your eczema plaques. Follow this twice a day for a month or until you begin to see improvement. Continue to take the capsules on a daily basis albeit at a reduced dose of 1-2 capsules per day.

EYE INFECTIONS

Medical definition
One of the most common and very contagious eye infections is conjunctivitis. Also known as pink eye, it is usually accompanied by a thick, yellow discharge, often crusting the eyes shut in the morning. Pink eye can be viral or bacterial in nature. The same type of virus that causes an upper-respiratory condition usually causes it.

Other conditions of the eye include Meibomian or tarsal cysts, caused by blockage of the duct, a stye or hordeolum, an infection of the root of the lash and Blepharitis, a chronic inflammation of the margin of the lids, and can lead to recurrent infections.

Treatment regimen
Take two capsules of allicin powder daily. Allicin liquid can be applied to a piece of lint and dabbed gently onto the infected area, being careful not to get any in the eye.

Testimonial
In July I had a very bad eye infection. I went to the doctors and was prescribed an eye ointment called "Brolene". I had to apply this morning and evening, and was told by the doctor if there was no improvement, to go back to the surgery. The day after applying Brolene my eyes had a sticky residue. Using salty water I had a battle to separate my eye lashes. After a couple of days my eyes were still red and sore. The doctor then prescribed an antibiotic eye cream. I had to apply two drops morning and evening. If no better, I was to go back to my doctor. Two creams later and there was still no

improvement. By this time I was really fed up. I then tried the allicin capsules taking two per day for two days. On the first day the itchiness had stopped and the redness became less. Then on the second day my eyes were completely clear. I was so impressed that I have told friends and work colleagues about your product. As I myself, after taking them for two days the difference was unbelievable. As soon as friends mention they've got a pain or a sniffle they are all quite keen to try anything, and I think they too have been very surprised by the results.
Thank you again. Yours sincerely,
Mrs C Francis, Sussex, England.

FOOD POISONING
(See DIARRHOEA and TRAVELLER'S TUMMY)

FUNGAL NAIL DISEASE

Medical definition
This is incredibly common in the Western World and in particular the United States where many millions of people suffer in silence. Caused by *Dermatophytes* and *Candida albicans* the fungus invades the toe or finger nails feeding off the rich supply of keratin found deep in the nail beds.

A number of factors will increase the likelihood of developing nail fungus, and these include poor hygiene, sugary diet, application of artificial nails and nail polish. Sadly yeast infections like this can often start from within our body so it is important to use an agent like allicin that can heal from within as well as treat the condition from without.

Treatment regimen
Simply apply a small dab of allicin cream to the skin around each infected nail or, if the fungus is on your fingernails, then add just 1 drop of allicin liquid to each nail twice daily. One other sensible action would be to prevent a recurrent infection by taking allicin capsules regularly (2 per day). Another interesting benefit from applying the liquid to fingernails is that it makes them much stronger and far less likely to crack or split. Apply just one drop per nail before you add your colour and within a few weeks you will notice a significant difference to the quality of your nails.

GINGIVITIS

Medical definition
Inflammation of the gums caused by plaque on the surfaces of the teeth at their necks. The gums are swollen and bleed easily. This can lead to periodontal disease but is reversible with good oral hygiene.

The composition of the plaque, which causes gingivitis, is a number of bacterial species. Gums are growing tissue, which require a consistent supply of nutrients for continued good health. Once the gums begin to degenerate a number of pockets can develop where food particles can accumulate and act as a magnet for further bacterial overgrowth – which also leads to the release of a wide range of toxins that continue the cycle of decay. Allicin powder can be easily placed on a number of foodstuffs to be chewed in the mouth and help to remove the various bacterial strains that infect our oral cavities.

Treatment regimen
Break open 2 allicin powder capsules per day and place the powder over your favourite food product and chew in your mouth twice daily – this will help to cleanse your mouth of bacteria.

HAY FEVER

Medical definition
Hay fever is an allergic reaction to airborne pollen from trees, grasses and other plants characterised by inflammation of the membrane lining the nose and sometimes the conjunctiva.

There are approximately 12 million sufferers of hay fever in the UK and more than 75 million in the USA. Symptoms vary from mild discomfort to those that are so severe that the sufferer cannot even go outdoors. One of the most recent peer reviewed studies that I have performed was looking at hay fever prevention and treatment with allicin powder capsules.

Treatment regimen
A daily dose of just 2 capsules per day can dramatically reduce the number of hay fever attacks that sufferers are likely to experience.

Testimonial
This really is quite amazing. For the first time ever I have been able to go about my normal routine without sneezing and constantly feeling blocked up. This allicin product is definitely the best thing I have ever used for treating my hay fever. Thanks ever so much.
Zoe M, Crawley Sussex.

HEAD LICE

Medical definition
Lice are a form of insect parasite that live only on the hairy parts of the body, different varieties being closely adapted to certain areas and races, even to the extent of having specially shaped claws to cling to the hair of different races.

The eggs of the head louse are found around the nape of the neck as small grey nits attached to the hair about halfway along and these take about two weeks to hatch, so the treatment must be repeated after a fortnight as only the lice are killed.

Control of infections with head lice has traditionally been performed using conventional insecticides rotated to avoid the development of resistance. In certain parts of the world the selection of strains of lice that have developed resistance to one or more insecticides. These "conventional" agents are also highly inflammable and rather toxic to the human body – their suitability for use on children is questionable. Faced with product claims that can no longer be wholly justified, an increasing number of consumers are experimenting with untested methods. A number of formulators have also decided to market products that are neither adequately tested for safety or efficacy nor are licensed for this application. Some materials used in this application are potentially toxic and, because many of the formulations are inappropriate, they may encourage the development of resistance to some of the potentially available alternative active substances.

Treatment regimen

Take a normal scoop of your favourite shampoo and add 20 drops of allicin liquid. Mix thoroughly and then shampoo the hair as normal. Like a conditioner leave the shampoo on for a couple of minutes and then wash off and repeat again. One bottle of allicin liquid will give you at least 11 treatments. This procedure should be repeated every day for a week. This will ensure that the eggs and nits are removed. At the same time you must use all the normal measures recommended by Public Health experts. So please ensure that you treat everyone in the family and that you comb out thoroughly any shells or eggs or dead lice that may still be stuck to the hair. At the end of the week your child's hair should be clean and nit free but it is probably worthwhile using this technique once or twice for the following two weeks to try to prevent a re-infestation as you can bet that somebody at school won't be as thorough a you! We have used this regimen at home on both our daughters with great success.

IMPETIGO

Medical definition

Impetigo is a superficial bacterial infection of the skin caused by *Staphylococcus aureus* infection. It mainly affects young children and is highly infectious, causing a yellow brown crusting on the skin.

For a young child this can be a particularly distressing condition as friends have to be warned "do not touch" as it is so infectious. Once again the bacterial species involved are *Staphylococcus,* which are highly sensitive to allicin treatment.

Treatment regimen

For children under the age of 5 it is best to remove the powder from the capsule and spread the allicin over the child's favourite food or dissolve it in a juice drink. For older children you should gently apply 2 drops of allicin liquid every 4 hours and dose 4 allicin capsules per day until the outbreak subsides. If your child has contact with any friends as well as family members then everyone should take 1-2 capsules a day to prevent the infection from passing on.

Testimonial

A few weeks ago little Eric from Atlanta GA developed a nasty bout of impetigo. His mother was really worried as she couldn't get hold of any antibiotics to calm it down and they were having a BBQ that day with lots of his friends invited. "I really wanted something to help immediately and a friend said she had just purchased some allicin capsules and a small supply of liquid. We used it immediately on Eric and literally within a few hours the attack had subsided and his plaques began to clear up. We were naturally delighted and would recommend this to anyone else who suffers from this debilitating condition."
Francis

IRRITABLE BOWEL SYNDROME

Medical definition

This is a common condition in which recurrent abdominal pain with constipation and/or diarrhoea continues for years without any deterioration in general health. Although the cause is unknown it is generally accepted that stress, anxiety and a series of recurrent infections in the intestine all contribute.

Most doctors will now agree that people who suffer from a wide range of digestive problems are likely to have an imbalance in the quality and content of their intestinal flora. Our stomach contains many hundreds of bacterial species, some of which are aggressive to our digestive system but many that are absolutely necessary for maintaining a normal healthy functioning digestive system. When this balance is upset symptoms will occur and until the balance is reset many people will continue to suffer.

Allicin can be described as a Pre-biotic in that it possesses an ability to kill harmful digestive bacteria like *Salmonella* and *Escherichia coli*, but will leave healthy bacterial species like *Lactobacillus* and *Acidophilus* alone. This means that your own population of friendly bacteria can go about their business and continue to flourish and replicate without any problems from an over-population of nasty bugs. If you add a good quality probiotic (pick one that is multi-strain and offers as many friendly bacterial strains as possible) you will also add significantly to your friendly digestive population. Within a very short period of time you will notice that your bowel habits return to normal and that you can happily eat whatever you like.

Treatment regimen
Add 2-4 capsules of allicin plus a multi-strain probiotic to every meal.

Testimonial
Jenny B from Stone in Kent has never been able to digest certain foods, especially bread. Already a convert to allicin she added in a probiotic and follows the regimen detailed above. Within just a matter of days she was able to digest meals more easily and even bread stopped giving her stomach cramps and constipation.

MOLLUSCUM CONTAGIOSUM

Medical definition
This is a common disease of the skin, mainly affecting children. Characterised by papules less than 5mm in diameter, each with a central depression, the disease is caused by a pox virus (others in this group include *variola* responsible for smallpox and vaccinia which causes cowpox) and is spread by direct contact. Untreated, the papules will disappear within 2 years.

This is a very distressing disease found in children especially just starting pre-school they are very unpleasant and most doctors will say that you just have to let the disease run its natural course. Well not now we have allicin! Please read the testimonial below as it really sums up how good allicin can be.

Treatment regimen
Apply a few drops of allicin liquid using a cotton bud twice daily. Increase frequency of application if you do not see any progress after 10 days

Testimonial

Earlier this year I was told by our doctor that our daughter was suffering from Molluscum Contagiosum, a condition of the skin which causes wart-like spots which eventually (over a period of months or even years) turn into large and painful pustules which eventually burst, sometimes leaving behind a scar or pit. She was five years old at the time and we had first noticed some spots when she was only two. Gradually, over this time, they had spread from her trunk and arms to her legs, and particularly between her legs and around the genital area. They were causing her a great deal of discomfort and embarrassment and it was most distressing to hear from the doctor that there was absolutely no treatment for them as they were caused by a virus. We were told that although painful and unsightly, they were otherwise totally harmless and that they would disappear eventually. When I heard, through a friend, that it might be possible to treat them with garlic, I decided that anything was worth a try. Through the Garlic Information Centre, we were given a bottle of pure allicin liquid (a component of fresh garlic most associated with healing properties) and told to apply it to our daughter's spots twice a day with a cotton bud. After only three days there was a noticeable improvement, and after a week the spots had completely gone. We were absolutely thrilled and could hardly believe that allicin had worked so effectively and so quickly! I know from talking to other parents that Molluscum Contagiosum is common in young children. I would thoroughly recommend trying this treatment. It can do no harm and may work for others as it has for us!

Claudia Macpherson, UK

NAPPY RASH

Medical definition

A red skin rash, within the nappy area, is usually caused by chemical irritation (ammoniacal dermatitis) or infection with *Candida*. Ammoniacal dermatitis is caused by skin contact with a soiled nappy. The stool bacteria react with urine to form the irritant ammonia.

Allicin cream has the consistency and quality to be used as a nappy rash treatment. It contains 125ppm (parts per million) allicin and can kill fungal infections at a concentration as low as 1.7ppm!

PARASITES

Medical definition
Any living thing, that lives in or on another living organism. The parasite, which may spend all or only part of its existence with the host, obtains food and/or shelter from the host and contributes nothing to its welfare. Some parasites cause irritation and interfere with bodily functions. Others destroy host tissues and release toxins into the body, thus injuring health and causing disease.

Human parasites include fungi, bacteria, viruses, protozoa and worms, and can all be treated with allicin.

Treatment regimen
Take 6 allicin powder capsules every day for at least 1 month and then reduce this back down to 2 per day. At the same time take allicin liquid and dilute it with distilled water: 1 part allicin liquid to 1 part water and take this 3 times per day for at least 1 month.

PARONYCHIA

Medical definition
An inflamed swelling of the nail folds usually caused by infection with *Staphylococcus aureus*. Chronic paronychia usually occurs in those who habitually engage in wet work where a secondary infection is caused by *Candida albicans*.

Antibiotics are often prescribed but of course the bacterium is now multi-drug resistant and therefore requires an agent like allicin that can kill both a bacterial and fungal infection. These two particular organisms are the most sensitive to allicin liquid and powder formulations (ie they are easily destroyed by allicin).

Treatment regimen

Apply allicin liquid directly to the infected area – just a few drops per day will be needed. Take 2-4 allicin capsules every day to get rid of any systemic infection (this is very common with *Candida*) and continue to take them after the infection clears to prevent it from returning.

PEPTIC ULCER

Medical definition

This is a breach in the lining of the digestive tract caused by digestion of the mucosa by pepsin and acid. A peptic ulcer can be found in the oesophagus, the stomach, duodenum or jejunum.

Ulcers are extremely common and for many years the medical profession had been convinced that the main cause was an over production of stomach acid. However we now know that even people with low volumes of stomach acid can get ulcers and interestingly stomach cancer is actually very common in people who cannot produce ANY stomach acid (achlorhydria) at all.

Treatment regimen

You will need to take a relatively large dose of allicin over a 2-4 week period to prevent the release of urea and to enable the allicin to penetrate the protective lining of the stomach so as to seek and destroy the *Helicobacter* infection. Take 6-10 capsules every day, either all in one go or spread out over the day. If you are already on a course of antibiotics then this dose should be cut in half. However, if the combination doesn't clear the infection then try using just allicin at the increased dosage level.

PNEUMONIA

Medical definition
The two most common types of pneumonia are atypical pneumonia and bronchopneumonia. Symptoms include high fever, flushed, dry skin, uncontrollable shivering, aching, malaise and a cough with viscid sputum. Respiration is rapid and shallow and often painful.

Atypical pneumonia is often caused by viruses, chlamydia (such as those caught from birds in psittacosis), mycoplasma or the *Legionella bacillus* of Legionnaires disease. Atypical pneumonia also involves the nervous system and digestive tract to cause confusion, hallucinations and diarrhoea. Bronchopneumonia can result due to the invasion of a variety of organisms because of the lowered resistance of the body and the poor circulation through the lungs. The base of the lungs and the bronchi become slowly infected and collapse, leading to stupor, confusion and eventually peaceful death.

Treatment regimen
Take 10 capsules of allicin powder every day for at least 1 month and then reduce this gradually over the course of about three months. If symptoms persist continue with the higher dose.

PRE-ECLAMPSIA

Medical definition
Pre-Eclampsia is caused by a defect in the placenta, which joins mother and baby and supplies the baby with nutrients and oxygen from the mother's blood. It is potentially life-threatening to mother and baby if allowed to develop and progress undetected.

Pre-Eclampsia is marked by circulatory disturbances, including high blood pressure in the mother and growth problems in the baby.

Early work suggests that allicin may have a significant role to play in the prevention of Pre-Eclampsia and of course it is perfectly safe to take. This is in direct opposition to the use of pharmaceutical agents that can rarely be used in pregnancy for fear of a serious direct affect on the baby.

Treatment regimen

Just one capsule a day should be taken throughout the pregnancy but this can be doubled or tripled if the blood pressure starts to rise. Several mums with a history of pre-eclampsia have used allicin during pregnancy and have not reported any rise in blood pressure.

PROTOZOAL INFECTIONS

(See PARASITES)

PSORIASIS

Medical definition

Psoriasis is a chronic but treatable auto-immune skin disease experienced by an estimated 80 million people around the world.

Psoriasis can greatly affect self-esteem and overall quality of life. It can develop anywhere on the skin, though it usually appears on the scalp, knees, elbows and torso. It also may affect the nails and joints.

The exact causes of psoriasis are complex and not fully understood, but genetic traits leading to abnormalities in the body's response to infection are believed to be the underlying basis. A specialised type of white blood cell called a T cell has been identified as playing a key role in the inflammation that eventually leads to psoriasis plaques and related symptoms. These malfunctioning T cells travel to the surface of the skin, and start an inflammatory reaction in which skin cells multiply 7 to 12 times faster than normal. The end result is the formation of psoriatic plaques. Allicin treatment for psoriasis fights back by reaching far beneath the skin to halt this psoriatic process exactly where it starts – in the immune system.

Treatment regimen

Take 6 allicin powder capsules a day for two weeks. Reduce to 2 capsules for a further two weeks. As a maintenance dose take one capsule thereafter to help prevent further attacks.

RINGWORM

Medical definition

A fungal infection of the skin, scalp and nails, caused by dermatophyte *Microsporium trichophyton* and *Epidermaphyton*, which can affect animals and are usually the source of infections in humans. Ringworm can be spread by direct contact or by infected materials. Lesions are ring-like and cause intense itching. The commonest form is Athlete's foot. Ringworm can also affect the groin and thighs.

Treatment regimen

Use a few drops of allicin liquid added to your normal shampoo and use 2-3 times a week. At the same time take 2-4 capsules per day and this can be reduced down to 1 per day once you have got rid of the infection.

ROSACEA

Medical definition

A chronic inflammatory disease of the face in which the skin becomes abnormally flushed. It can become pustular and there may be associated keratinitis. Most common in women and the cause is now thought to be a type of parasite known as *Demodex*, which is found in the hair follicles and sebaceous glands. They resemble tiny worms and they are difficult to dislodge. It is also thought that the bacterium *Helicobacter pylori* may also be responsible for rosacea. Allicin will be able to destroy these parasites and bacterial infections.

Treatment regimen

Apply 1 or 2 drops of allicin liquid or cream directly to the pustules once or twice per day. Also add 2 allicin powder capsules per day permanently to boost your immune system.

SCABIES

Medical definition
This is a skin infection caused by the mite Sarcoptes scabiei, typified by severe itching, especially at night. Characteristic red papules are caused by deposits of faeces left by the mite, which tunnels into the skin to start laying eggs. New hatched mites are easily spread to other people by direct contact. Intense itching represents an allergic reaction to the mite, its eggs and faeces.

The penis, nipples and the skin between the fingers are the most commonly affected areas. Normal treatment is with insecticides including Lindane and all sexual contacts and family members must be treated.

Treatment regimen
Currently allicin has not been used to any great extent on treating scabies. However, as we have already seen, allicin can kill head lice so it would make sense to use the liquid in a soap to try and get rid of the mites. A soap formulation of allicin is recommended.

SHINGLES

Medical definition
This is another herpetic virus known as *Herpes Zoster.*

Chickenpox is the primary infection of this virus and it is only when this reactivates that it produces the condition known as shingles.

Treatment regimen
A large dose of allicin capsules, 6 to 10 per day should be taken for several months to try and remove this resistant infection.

SINUSITIS

Medical definition

Sinusitis is an inflammation of the sinus cavities and may be caused by a variety of factors. Most recently Johns Hopkins Medical School in America has shown that recurrent sinusitis is often associated with a fungal infection. Other contributory factors will include food allergy reactions and inhalant allergy from existing medications.

Worldwide millions of people suffer from sinus disease, which causes symptoms like hay fever, runny nose and post nasal drip. People are encouraged to buy expensive over the counter medications that may relieve symptoms for a short period. A minor operation to unplug the sinuses and remove all the infection built up is a relatively simple day surgery operation but rather uncomfortable. Unfortunately the symptoms usually recur after just a few months – since the fungal component of this infection keeps returning.

Treatment regimen

Take 1-3 capsules of allicin powder daily for 2 weeks followed by a maintenance dose of 1 capsule daily. You can also inhale the liquid formulation twice daily to add to the effect.

Testimonial

Mr JH from Bexhill, UK, Mr PD from Prescott, Arizona and Mrs JAH from Oslo, Norway all had recurrent and persistent sinusitis. Having also had an operation to unblock the sinus cavities they still had the common symptoms including sneezing, runny nose and a constant feeling of being bunged up. They all tried using allicin and adopted the above protocol and gained excellent benefits.

SORE THROAT

Medical definition

A condition caused by a variety of microbes including bacteria, virus and fungal species.

As one of the commonest infections known to man it is also one of the most troublesome, causing intense discomfort that hitherto could only be temporarily alleviated by anaesthetic lozenges bought over the counter.

TICK BORNE DISEASES

See PARASITE INFESTATIONS

THRUSH

See CANDIDA INFECTIONS

TOOTHACHE

Toothache is almost always caused by an infection. An infection can be easily treated with allicin powder or liquid. In ancient times people used to cut up a clove of garlic and place it in or around the tooth abscess. Pain relief was usually immediate.

Treatment regimen

Apply the liquid by rubbing a few drops in and around the painful area or alternatively open up a capsule and rub a little allicin powder over the infected area.

TRAVELLER'S TUMMY

Medical definition

Those who travel to different parts of the world are at increased risk of infection from organisms in the locality as well as from alterations to their diet. Traveller's tummy is a result of coming into contact with a strain of *E. coli* with which the gut is unfamiliar. Symptoms can vary; though normally include abdominal pain and diarrhoea.

The maxim that travel broadens the mind but loosens the bowels is all too true for up to half of us travelling to "high risk" areas such as South America, Asia, Africa and parts of the Middle East (*Drugs and Therapeutics Bulletin*, June 2002). The familiar symptoms of "the runs"and cramps, accompanied by nausea and/or vomiting, can be both embarrassing and distressing. Consuming food or drink contaminated with bacteria, viruses, or parasites is usually to blame for travellers' diarrhoea. Most cases are bacterial, with *E. coli* the prime suspect.

There are three approaches to coping with travellers' diarrhoea: prevention (for instance by taking allicin powder capsules and probiotics before you go to ward off infection); self-treatment (taking a self-treatment kit with you this would also include a fluid replacement); and letting it take its course. The choice depends largely on your age, your general health, and the type of holiday envisaged. Most bouts of travellers' diarrhoea clear up spontaneously in two to three days. But it's important to replace the fluid lost as dehydration can be dangerous, especially in the elderly and very young.

Aim for prevention if you have a condition that makes you prone to infection, for instance low immunity, diabetes, or an ailment that requires drugs to suppress stomach acid. In such cases it's probably worth discussing travel plans and the need for prophylactic antibiotics with your doctor but for most people, the US National Institutes of Health and the Centres for Disease Control advise against taking antibiotics for prevention of traveller's diarrhoea.

An alternative preventative approach is to take allicin powder capsules and a probiotic for a week before travelling. Trials have shown that probiotics can help restore the colonies of "friendly" bacteria that have been flushed out by infection and treatment and that allicin can both prevent bacterial infections and get rid of them quickly if you do pick one up.

If you choose the second option, self-treatment, there are several alternatives. Taking antibiotics after infection will usually shorten the duration of symptoms. Ciprofloxacin will deal with many of the culprit bugs but by adding allicin you get an extra benefit since the duration of the symptoms can be reduced to less than 6 hours, resistance won't be a problem as the allicin can wipe our resistant cipro bugs and of course the allicin has another advantage of being able to work against viral or parasitic infections as well.

You should consult a doctor if there's any visible blood or mucous in your stool, or if the diarrhoea persists for more than five days – diarrhoea can be the signal for several serious conditions such as cholera, typhoid and parasitic infections.

Treatment regimen
As well as following the usual safe practices appropriate to your destinations, start your course of allicin powder capsules and a probiotic 7 days before you travel, maintain it throughout your holiday and continue the course for 7 days after you return.

VERRUCAE (Plantar warts)

Medical definition
Plantar warts (verrucae) occur on the soles of the feet and are often contracted in warm moist areas, particularly swimming pools and showers.

Treatment regimen
Use allicin liquid after washing, once a day, until the warts disappear.

WARTS

Medical definition
A wart is a benign growth on the skin caused by infection with human *papillomavirus*. Common warts are firm horny papules, found mainly on the backs of the hands. Most will clear spontaneously within 2 years. Plane warts are flat and skin colored and therefore difficult to see; they are usually found on the face and may be present in very large numbers. Genital warts are frequently associated with other genital infections and affected women have an increased risk of developing cervical cancer.

Treatment regimen and Testimonial

Apply allicin cream or liquid once or twice daily by massaging a small amount into the surface of the wart. Users report that the treatment takes effect in approximately 2 weeks and the warts have completely disappeared within 1 month. One user re-applied allicin every day for no more than a week and found the warts had completely disappeared.

WOUNDS

Medical definition

A break in the structure of an organ or tissue caused by an external agent.

Current research shows that allicin formulations can help to heal wounds quickly and prevent infection.

Treatment regimen

If an infection is present in a wound then allicin liquid, backed up by a normal dose of allicin powder capsules does appear to remove stubborn wound infections.

Personal Testimonial

The author writes: "I am a bit clumsy and have to admit that just about every time I am out in the backyard I do something that causes me a minor injury! Well now I routinely apply a little allicin liquid to the bandaid before I stick it over the wound. A short while ago I got a nasty wooden splinter in my thumb – it immediately began to swell and was very painful. I managed to get the wood out but my thumb was beginning to balloon. So I just applied 2 drops of allicin liquid to the plaster and repeated this a few hours later. The pain had already gone and within a day the swelling was much better and I healed perfectly. This is also unusual for me as I am a diabetic and am very slow to heal. So this time my thumb healed perfectly the old skin flaked away to reveal a perfectly healed wound with no scarring. I could have used a small dose of powder as an alternative but allicin liquid is really easy to use."

Part Two
Chapter Five...

More serious conditions where allicin has been shown to be helpful

The conditions described in the previous chapter can be self-treated using allicin quite safely, although it must be re-emphasised that where a treatment is being prescribed by a doctor, whether it be ongoing or short-term, you should always defer to that advice and, if you decide to treat yourself with allicin, discuss what you are planning with your practitioner.

There are, of course, a range of medical conditions, which are of a more serious nature where there are indications that allicin has a part to play. I feel it prudent to offer the following as no more than an indication of the state of play:

AIDS (Acquired Immunodeficiency Syndrome)

Medical definition
A syndrome first identified in Los Angeles in 1981; a description of the causative virus – the human immunodeficiency virus (HIV) – was available in 1983 the virus destroys a subgroup in lymphocytes, resulting in suppression of the body's immune response. AIDS is essentially a sexually transmitted disease, either homosexually or heterosexually. The two other main routes of spread are via infected blood or blood products and by the maternofoetal route.

For those people who do enter a chronic stage there may be illness of varying severity including persistant generalised involvement of the lymph nodes – this is termed ARC (AIDS Related Complex) including intermittent fever, weight loss, diarrhoea, fatigue and night sweats. Often opportunistic infections can be life threatening to AIDS sufferers, especially pneumonia caused by the protozoan (*Pneumocystis Carinii*) and possible tumors leading to Karposi's Sarcoma. Thus, it is not actually the AIDS virus that kills, but the infections that are easily picked up by having a seriously depleted immune system.

With this in mind it is clear that large doses of allicin powder can help to prevent infections from developing in HIV and sero-converted AIDS sufferers. By boosting the immune system and destroying a wide range of infectious organisms allicin powder can definitely help.

In the USA, trials in AIDS patients have demonstrated enhancement of natural killer cell activity using garlic extracts and Chinese studies with viral infections in bone marrow transplant patients have demonstrated a "potent antiviral activity". Human population studies have shown that regular intake reduces the risk of oesophageal, stomach and colon cancer. This was thought to be due to the antioxidant effect of allicin in reducing the formation of carcinogenic compounds in the gastro-intestinal tract.

Testimonial

As this book went to press David from New York City had been HIV+ for 10 years and has had full-blown AIDS for 2 years. He picked up a serious infection and used large doses of allicin powder capsules to get rid of this infection:

As someone who has had full-blown AIDS for over two years, I can attest to the strength and promise of allicin powder capsules. For a quick example, I was experiencing diarrhoea about once every day or two – and then I started taking the capsules. Since I started using them, I have not had diarrhoea ONCE. I have been using allicin powder capsules for about two months now. More dramatically, when I received my first shipment in the mail, I had been sick for three days with a viral infection and had been feeling worse each day. On the third day, I was really quite miserable and ill, especially realising that this illness could go on for two or three weeks – or worse. I started taking my first capsule toward the end of that third day, and two days later (Superbowl Sunday evening in the US), I was sitting up, eating a pizza, and enjoying watching television. I was surprised that I felt so much better in such a relatively short (48 hours) period of time. By the end of the third day I felt like I was basically over my viral infection, and that the "bug" had been killed. Naturally, I was not back to full vigor just yet, but each day, on allicin capsules, I felt stronger, healthier and more vigorous. I was back to my full strength and vigor in about ten days, which is about what it would be for anyone. I was astounded at the healing power that allicin apparently contains. I feel like allicin will, in time, prove itself to be, essentially an "immune system in pill form", seemingly without any drawbacks, side effects etc. The potential for improved health for humankind could – based on my own personal experience – be enormous, truly staggering.

If allicin could offer this kind of powerful help to someone in my condition, what could it do for people with normal immune systems? Since I've started using this product, I have not experienced any other abnormal health problems at all, and I'm not taking any other medicines. I'm now beginning to think that I may be able to "get my life back", return to work etc. This – as opposed to thinking that my days were more or less "numbered"! I now once again do things that I enjoy – with confidence – for I no longer feel afraid to over-exert myself physically, etc. My life has, relatively speaking, "gone back to normal". I consider allicin powder capsules to be a medical miracle.

A few weeks later David sent me another letter:

More good news – after years of having "borderline-high" blood pressure, my last visit to the doctor tells me my blood pressure is "good"! At first I thought, "How could that be possible? Why would my blood pressure suddenly be so different?" I think it's the allicin. I can't think of any other change in my life that might have lowered my blood pressure to such a degree.

BACTERIAL INFECTIONS

Medical definition

A group of microorganisms, all of which lack a distinct nuclear membrane and are considered to be more primitive than animal, plant or human cells. Most bacteria are single celled.

Bacteria reproduce asexually by simple division of cells and incomplete separation of daughter cells can lead to the formation of colonies consisting of different numbers and arrangements of cells all with different and complex shapes. Bacteria are very widely distributed. Some live in soil, water or air; others are parasites of man, animals and plants and many cause disease by producing toxins.

The minimum inhibitory concentration of allicin in parts per million for some common bacterial species

• Streptococcus pyogenes	16 ppm	(flesh eating bacteria)
• Staphylococcus aureus	16 ppm	(implicated in eczema)
• Listeria monocytogenes	16 ppm	(often caught from animals)
• Escherichia Coli 0157	32 ppm	(poorly cooked meat)
• Salmonella typhimurium	32 ppm	(raw eggs)
• Clostridium perfringens	64 ppm	(animals and man)
• Helicobacter pylori	16 ppm	(stomach ulcers)
• Yersinia enterocolitica	12 ppm	(stomach upsets)
• Bacillus subtilus	<3 ppm	(causes conjunctivitis)

Case study - drug-resistant *Streptococcus*

In Norway Camilla, a young Mother of 2 children went into hospital to have her third child by caesarian section. Although everything went well she picked up an infection, a not uncommon event in even the best-run hospitals. Camilla had a drug resistant *streptococcus* and after she was discharged her wound failed to heal for several months and she had a systemic infection that made her tired, washed out and unable to look after her new baby or the family. With her husband taking time off work Camilla was desperate. Then she read about allicin. After taking 10 capsules per day for 4 weeks she began to feel better. Although she had already stopped taking the antibiotics in less than a month her specimens came back negative – no bacterial infection. No bacteria found in her throat, her underarms or her vagina. She was clear, healthy and cured.

CANCER

Medical definition

Cancer is a disease of metabolic imbalance and can originate in a thousand different ways. Cancer occurs when cells lose their ability to replicate in an orderly fashion, they divide too rapidly and grow without any order. Too much tissue is produced and tumors begin to form. Tumors can be either benign or malignant.

Malignant tumors can invade and destroy nearby tissue and organs. Cancer cells can spread to other parts of the body and form new tumors.

It is estimated that one in three people will develop a type of cancer at some time in their life and that cancer continues to account for around 25 per cent of all deaths recorded each year. Traditional Chinese medicine has always used garlic as a part of any treatment for the patients who suffered from a tumor or cancer. The search for compounds that prevent cancer has intensified with the mounting evidence that many types of cancer are caused or triggered by factors relating to lifestyle and environment. It is well documented that allicin can strengthen the immune system, which is vitally important for fighting cancer. When I reviewed this important area of medicine I was surprised and pleased to find a considerable amount of data already published indicating that by taking allicin powder capsules regularly you can confer some degree of protection against various stomach cancers, boost your CD4-T cell count and convey some degree of protection.

Interestingly, the medical community has known about this for years and is currently trying to establish which compounds are the most protective, since evidence also shows major benefits from diallyl disulphide, which is a common breakdown component of allicin powder. Many of the breakdown products from allicin have been tested for their inhibiting effect on cancer cells and in most experiments inhibition of tumor growth was established.

Researchers concluded that evidence from laboratory experiments and population surveys is presently not conclusive as to the preventative activity of allicin. However, they also indicated that the available evidence warrants further research into the possible role of allicin in the prevention of cancer in humans.

Anti-cancer effects

In ancient times, garlic was used for the treatment of cancer of the uterus. Numerous reports, including several important epidemiological studies, have entered the scientific literature ever since, asserting that garlic has a favourable effect on various forms of cancer. The following provides an overview of the current research and points of view concerning this very interesting special area of medicine:

Six decades ago, several statistical studies indicated that cancer occurs the least in those countries where garlic and onions are eaten regularly - for instance, in the Provence region of France, Italy, the Netherlands, the Balkans, Egypt, India, and China. A review article, published in 1936, referred to the connection between nutrition and cancer, and especially to the cancer growth-inhibiting effect of leek plants (*Allium* plants). The practicing physicians of the time were very good observers but knew almost nothing about the scientific background to this phenomenon.

It was thought that the inhibitory action of garlic on putrefaction in the intestines, together with the secretion-stimulating effect, brought about detoxification and an increase in resistance. Stimulation of gastric juice secretion and restoration of the intestinal flora, combined with the resulting prevention of gastrointestinal autointoxication, may help to remove at least one of the possible causes of cancer. Garlic was therefore thought to have potential as a cancer preventative agent. More recently, this idea has again been pursued, not only in Europe, but also in the Third World countries, where the favourable effects of garlic for cancer are well known. For instance, the consumption of black or green tea, as well as of garlic, is known to be a culinary practice, which inhibits tumorigenesis in the lung, forestomach, and oesophagus.

The only known study in which garlic has been used to treat patients with advanced stages of cancer was conducted by Spivak (1962). An aqueous garlic juice preparation was administered in doses of 0.2-2mL intravenously or 1-5mL intramuscularly daily for 3-7 days. Of 35 patients with cancer at various sites (lung, cervix, stomach, lower lip, mammary gland, larynx, and leukemia), 26 showed positive treatment results of differing degrees, though complete healing was not achieved in any case. There is a single-case report, however, of a man whose pituitary tumour shrank by 50 per cent during the 5 months in which he ate 5-7 grams of fresh garlic daily. This was the first case ever reported of reduction of this type of tumor without chemotherapy or surgery.

Some notable success stories have been reported using allicin powder capsules. Especially in Norway where patients with various types of cancer have dramatically improved their CD4-T cell count (remember this is a measure of how efficient your immune system is) – patients going through chemotherapy or radiotherapy tend to have very poorly functioning immune systems since they are effectively destroyed by treatment.

Anti-cancer Effects: Active Compounds

From the many publications that have just been reviewed, it is apparent that the anti-cancer effects of garlic are likely due, perhaps equally, to allicin and allicin-derived compounds as well as unidentified compounds not related to allicin. The following is a summary of the evidence for possible active compounds.

1. Epidemiological studies from six different countries have consistently shown that garlic consumption is associated with decreased risk of gastrointestinal cancer. Since garlic is mainly eaten cooked (alliinase inactivated) in most of these countries, allicin is unlikely to be the cause of significant gastrointestinal cancer reduction.

2. A major decrease in incidence of gastric cancer in China, particularly where large amounts of allicin-yielding fresh garlic are eaten, is associated with the antibiotic effects of garlic and its thiosulfinates (allicin) toward decreasing the amount of nitrate-reducing bacteria in the stomach and hence the amounts of carcinogenic nitrosamines formed. Therefore, allicin does appear to have an important role in prevention of gastric cancer.

3. Animal studies have indicated the importance of allicin, since dietary fresh garlic, but not alliinase-inhibited garlic, greatly decreased breast cancer incidence in C3H mice.

A large number of animal studies with allicin-derived Diallyl disulphide and Diallyl sulphide, most using very large doses (100-200mg/kg) have shown positive effects toward decreasing carcinogen-induced cancer. Although allicin itself has not been tested, these studies indicate that allicin-derived compounds have the ability to affect cancer incidence.

HEPATITIS

Medical definition

This is inflammation of the liver and can be caused by viruses, toxic substances or immunological abnormalities. There are many different types, some transmitted sexually and others through an exchange of body fluids from an infected person.

Hepatitis is very difficult to treat and every year in America alone 400,000 people develop a Hepatitis B or C infection. Many of the viruses that can cause hepatitis are from the herpetic family and will also include Epstein-Barr type viral infections. We already know that allicin has the ability to destroy and prevent these organisms from flaring up in the human body. So allicin formulations will have some benefit but the complexity and very nature of hepatitis make this difficult to show results. However the natural boost to the immune system that allicin can give will have some beneficial activity.

MRSA INFECTION (Methicillin Resistant *Staphylococcus Aureus*)

Medical definition

The bacteria Methicillin Resistant *Staphylococcus Aureus* (MRSA) and several other strains of bacteria live in our gut, known as 'alert organisms' (also called gentamicin resistant organisms). In most cases these bacteria cause no problems but when they enter another body system, such as the blood or urine, they may cause illness.

When colonised, people that are carrying the bacteria in their nose, throat or gut, or on their skin do not show any symptoms. However, if the patient has a temperature, and or redness of a wound this may indicate an infection.

These bacteria are resistant to most conventional antibiotics.

Patients now get released from hospital too soon, even before wounds have properly healed. Speaking with my own doctor recently he could name 8 patients in our local area who had a resistant MRSA infection at home trying deparately to get rid of it.

One such person was Deborah whose experience her mother reports below.

Testimonial

Her (Deborah's) wounds are on her spine. One close to the top, which is approx.2cm by 1.5cm this is overgranulated and weeps. The other is approx. 0.75cm by 0.5cm and near her waistline this is overgranulated but only weeps a little. She had a major spinal operation two years ago and although she has had antibiotics through a Hickman line and a wash-out so far nothing has worked. She has been on oral antibiotics and creams for several months but nothing has been able to shift the MRSA infection. The only option available to her via the hospital is to have all the metalwork removed. As you can imagine she does not want to go back into hospital nor does she want the metalwork removed. We would be very grateful if you could produce a cream and some capsules for her. If you require any further information we can speak to the District Nurses on Saturday, as she dresses her wounds then, whilst I do them during the week.

Just a few weeks later

Dear Peter

I had not been in touch as mum said she had emailed you. I don't think she wanted to get carried away, but the news is very exciting - I no longer have any infection in my back and it is all thanks to the treatments you so generously suggested. Having had these two wounds on my back weeping for 2 years I don't know quite how to thank you and hope that I get the opportunity to thank you in person at some point. I will also be telling anyone who may benefit from allicin how miraculous it is.

I am going to the hospital on Thursday. I am not sure if my consultant can quite believe what has happened, as he, along with some of my district nurses, are not too happy about the thought of using alternative remedies. When I think how many courses of antibiotics I have been instructed to take in the last 2 years and how many biopsies came back positive for MRSA, I am not surprised that the medical staff cannot believe it!

Thank you once again for all you have done. You saved me from another horrendous operation. Maybe I can repay you in some way. For instance, if it would be of any benefit, I could write something about my experience with MRSA and how allicin cured it, if that might help promote the product - just a thought.
Yours eternally grateful
Deborah

SARS (Severe Acute Respiratory Syndrome)

Medical definition

The symptoms of SARS are a lot like pneumonia or the flu. People get a very high fever - at least 100.4 degrees. They also usually have shortness of breath or other problems breathing and a dry cough. Some people get other symptoms including a headache, stiff or achy muscles, and a loss of appetite, fatigue, a rash and diarrhoea.

Doctors believe that it is spread primarily by tiny droplets that get airborne when someone sneezes or coughs, or by contact with other bodily fluids such as blood and faeces. Most people who have contracted SARS outside of Asia have either recently travelled to Asian countries where it was spreading or had close contact with someone who recently returned from there or became infected by someone who travelled there.

The disease is caused by a microbe known as a *coronavirus*. *Coronaviruses* usually just cause the common cold, but can cause serious respiratory illnesses in animals.

Antibiotics don't seem to work, which is usually the case with virus-caused diseases.

All allicin formulations, that is powder, liquid and cream, have been requisitioned in America for testing by The National Institute for Health (NIH), the National Institute for Allergy and Infectious Diseases (NIAID) and The United States Army Military Research Institute for Infectious Diseases (USAMRIID). They are performing tests against a wide range of microbial species including SARS, West Nile Virus, EEE (Eastern Equine Encephalitis), Smallpox, Vaccinia and Variola species.

TUBERCULOSIS

Medical definition

An infectious disease caused by the bacterium *Mycobacterium tuberculosis*, formerly known as consumption or wasting disease.

Mycobacterium tuberculosis (TB) can lay dormant for many years, but chronic infection is spread very easily by coughing or sneezing. Unfortunately TB is once again on the increase as the number of cases reported in major international cities has more than doubled in the last 5 years. This is partly due to the influx of refugees and asylum seekers from parts of the world where TB is endemic.

It is reported that London is the TB capital of Europe and New York has set up special hospitals just to treat resistant cases. What is worrying though is a report broadcast on National Geographic TV Channel that in Russia 4 million people are infected with TB, many of which are carrying drug resistant strains who are just walking the streets spreading the pool of infection. Unfortunately a large number of Russian prisoners are also infected and do not qualify for any treatment. So when they are released they are then able to spread the disease still further.

Recently a number of strains of MDR TB were isolated from patients in a London teaching hospital. The patients are often treated by combinations of antibiotics including Streptomycin and Rifampicin. Any growth in the presence of an antimicrobial is significant with MDR *Mycobacterium tuberculosis* and growth was noted on all cases where strains from these patients were treated with Streptomycin. However no growth was found where strains were treated with allicin liquid.

All strains isolated were completely killed off by allicin liquid. Since *Mycobacterium tuberculosis* tends to present mostly in the lungs we would expect allicin formulations to work very well. This is because allicin has a propensity for the lung tissue, as it is very useful in chest infections and other diseases of the lung like asthma. Aside from this allicin will boost the immune system substantially and allow your body to begin fighting off this serious infection.

Treatment regimen
Begin by taking allicin liquid several times a day. Dilute allicin liquid 1 part allicin to 2 parts water and take 10ml (two teaspoons full) every day. Add 6 capsules of allicin powder daily and continue this routine for a period of several weeks until any progress is noted.

Part Three...

The Future

In the last three decades we have seen several viral and bacterial epidemics take place at a time when we would have expected the eradication of many infectious diseases. Some people say this is due to the over-use of too-potent antibiotics, which eliminate protective infecting agents. Others believe it might be the widespread use of vaccines. There are even conspiracy theorists who believe they may be the results of terrorist acts or leakage of viral mutants from research laboratories.

Whatever the cause, globalisation and the increasing availability of long distance flights - Shanghai to Toronto for example - is making the spread of infections around the world much easier.

In the 21st Century we have already identified a number of infectious organisms that can and will present a major problem to patients, physicians, health care workers and administrators the world over.

These include MRSA, MDR Tuberculosis, VRE *Vancomycin resistant enterococcus*, VRSA – *Vancomycin resistant Staphylococcus aureus*, VISA and GISA (*Glycopeptide intermediate resistant Staphylococcus aureus*). All these have proven to be sensitive to allicin and a sixth, PRSP Penicillin resistant *Streptococcus pneumonia*, although not yet tested, is very likely to be.

With MRSA now reported in the "healthy community" the writing is already on the wall. We need something that can take on these superbugs. We need to reduce our dependence on pharmaceutical antibiotics, or at least make them more effective, by reducing the extent to which they are used.

By not doing that, these powerful microbes will take over. Already infectious disease is a bigger killer than heart disease or cancer. The species above cannot be treated by anything the pharmaceutical industry has to offer – even the latest antibiotics, yet to reach the market, are unable to kill certain species of bacteria. We have seen international panic over SARS and MRSA spreading. This is bad enough but it is really quite worrying when you realise that doctors routinely encounter organisms like *E. coli, Helicobacter pylori, Tuberculosis, Herpes virus, Acinetobacter, Cryptosporidium, Campylobacter,* HIV, *Salmonella, Cholera, Streptococcus Pyogenes* flesh eating bacteria and others that are becoming multi drug resistant.

It is estimated that the number of bacteria, virus and fungal pathogens to be found either in or around every human being is so large as to be virtually infinite. This is why still, after 70 years of producing pharmaceutical antibiotics, recent surveys indicate that 90 percent of visits to doctor's surgeries are infection related. It is also why more than one million metric tons of antibiotics have been dispersed into the biosphere in the past 50 years – half for human use and half for animal use which means that the indigenous bacteria of all living species are richly populated with resistant bacteria that we cannot get rid of. Is it any wonder that public health physicians are worried?

Why are we losing the battle?

Recent reports indicate that bacteria may send messages to each other about resisting antibiotic poisoning (*Medicine Today*, June 2002). In fact, bacterial signalling is going on all the time, all over your body, but especially in your mouth and guts. Finding ways of interfering with this signalling process is the latest objective of researchers who are waging the antibiotic arms race.

A major result of these bacterial conversations are bacterial communities! Among the more extraordinary sights visible through the latest confocal laser scanning microscopes, which allows objects to be viewed almost in 3D, are what have been dubbed "slime cities" – armoured defensive communities where bacteria live and reproduce, safe from antibiotics, your immune system and other predators.

Known technically as biofilms, they are currently the target of intense research because it is becoming increasingly clear that they are at the root of some of our most intractable conditions. The American Centres for Disease Control and Prevention estimate that 65 percent of human bacterial infections involve biofilms. Not only are they responsible for tooth decay and gum disease but they also cause many of the problems associated with cystic fibrosis, ear infections and infections of the prostate gland and the heart. They cause an estimated $6 billion a year of expenditure in the USA by causing hard-to-treat infections on catheters, artificial heart valves and other medical implants.

Similarly, irrational prescribing causes over-use of the very agents used to remove these infectious organisms. It is estimated that every year in the States, 10 million adults seek treatment for acute bronchitis and most are given antibiotics, even though the pathogens involved in most cases are viruses, which antibiotics aren't designed to work on.

We tend to think of bacteria as primitive single cell creatures, but when they are organised into a biofilm they differentiate, communicate, cooperate and deploy collective defences against antibiotics. In short, they behave like a multicellular organism.

In fact, bacteria from biofilms were among the first ever to be seen through a microscope when pioneer Antony van Leeuwenhoek looked at plaque – a biofilm – scraped from his own teeth in the late 1600's. But it wasn't until the 1970's that scientists began to appreciate just how complex these micro slime cities are. Plaque, for instance, is founded on a base of dense opaque slime about 5 micrometres thick. Above this, vast colonies of bacteria shaped like mushrooms or cones rise to between 100 to 200 micrometres.

Enclosed within their highly effective defensive wall of slime live communities of a variety of bacterial strains. One researcher described them thus: "The 'cities' are permeated at all levels by a network of channels through which water, bacterial garbage, nutrients, enzymes, metabolites and oxygen travel to and fro.

"The bacteria inside a biofilm, comprising 15 percent bacterial cells and 85 percent slime, are 1000 times less likely to succumb to antibiotics than bacteria in free-floating state"

The notion that bacteria can talk to each other was first proposed more than 30 years ago by scientists studying "glow in the dark" bacteria, such as *Vibro fischeri*, that live in the specialised "light organs" of certain squid and marine fish. The bacteria don't glow as individuals swimming freely, but when enough of them form a group, their illuminations are switched on. So they must have some way of letting each other know when enough of them have gathered. However, it wasn't until the 1980's that researchers identified the chemical they each put out – AHL (acyl-homoserine lactone). The more of them there are in one place, the higher the level of AHL. Above a certain threshold the concentration of AHL triggers the luminescence, in a mechanism usually referred to as Quorum Sensing.

But gradually a better understanding of just how biofilms fight off antibiotics is emerging. The bacteria benefit from pooling their effects. For instance, in a biofilm some bacteria can produce an enzyme that inactivates the antiseptic hydrogen peroxide, but a single bacterium can't make enough to save itself. Another factor is that even if an antibiotic does get through and kill off some bacterial inhabitants, a substantial number are likely to survive. This is because bacteria exist in a spectrum of physiological states from rapidly growing to dormant. Antibiotics usually target some activity like cell division, and that means that the dormant ones will usually live to fight another day.

Dr Richard Novick has found that *Staphylococcus aureus* can be divided into four different types, each with slightly different signalling molecules. The molecules used by one type stimulated activity in its own group but inhibited it in the others – an example of the way bacteria compete with each other. This particular bacterium is a worry to virtually every health-care establishment in the Western World as it has developed a number of strains that are resistant to all pharmaceutical antibiotics, even Vancomycin, a toxic parenteral drug usually reserved as a last resort.

Bacteria are sufficiently well organised to be able to find ways of avoiding the immune system. For instance, in *Vibrio cholerae*, the bacterium that causes cholera, the same genes involved in regulating quorum sensing also turn on the toxin production (*Proc Natl Acad Sci*, 5 March 2002). The value of this strategy is that a few toxic bacteria might alert the immune system and be rapidly engulfed. By waiting to turn on toxicity until there are enough of them, they have a better chance of overwhelming the host's defences.

> "It has been estimated that 40 percent of proteins in bacterial walls are different in "slime city dwellers" from those that are "free ranging". The implication of this is that some of the proteins identified in cultures and targeted by antibiotics simply aren't there in city dwellers"

Most of the work on quorum sensing has concentrated on chemicals that allow members of the same species to talk to one another. However, while Dr Bonnie Bassler at Princeton University was working on the luminous bacteria that led to the finding of quorum sensing in the first place, she made the remarkable discovery that signals from other bacteria could also turn on their lights. It seems that bacteria have some sort of Esperanto – a common language (*Nature*, 31 January 2002) – which involves a protein known as A1-2. Exactly what this system is used for isn't clear yet. However, among the bacteria that infect humans, those found to produce A1-2 include *Escherichia coli* (food poisoning), *Haemophilus influenzae* (pneumonia and meningitis), *Helicobacter pylori* (peptic ulcers), *Yersinia pestis* (bubonic plague) and *Staphylococcus aureus* (pneumonia, meningitis and toxic shock syndrome).

> "ALL of these bacteria can be killed by low concentrations of allicin"

Allicin, mother nature's defender, is an agent that can break up a biofilm, destroy a wide range of bacterial species, wipe out fungal infections, boost an under active immune system, reduce cholesterol and blood pressure levels, prevent viral infections, kill off parasites, remove protozoal organisms, vasodilate when necessary, prevent the release of histamine, and even prevent mosquitoes from attacking – yes all of this from an agent that can be produced from fresh garlic!

Work is currently underway, using the latest technology, to allow us to blast apart a bacterial cell and detect exactly which proteins and enzymes it can produce. Then the same species is treated with allicin liquid or powder, blasted apart again and analysed to see which proteins and enzymes have been disabled and which, therefore, are inactive and unable to infect us. We already know that allicin is capable of penetrating bacterial cell walls and preventing the release of many enzymes that are toxic to humans. Allicin formulations are also effective against a wide spectrum of bacterial species, viral infections, fungal and protozoal disease as well as a large number of parasite problems.

Part Four...

Little known facts and tips about Garlic

Since garlic dates back many centuries, there are an accumulation of facts and tips. These are covered in the following pages and give details about garlic's uses in cooking, the garden and animals.

Figures and facts are shown for quantities of consumption, the make up of garlic and there are even some more light-hearted details included, which we don't take too seriously now, such as the attribution of garlic to Vampires!

There are lots of details for use in health and wellbeing, especially in relation to the heart and blood pressure. Garlic has been proven to help, but remember before trying out any of these little tips, consult a healthcare practitioner if you are taking medication.

So, do you know?...

Garlic around the globe

The World consumption of garlic per year is approximately 1 clove for every living person!

In 1992 the world crop of garlic was estimated by the United Nations as 2,315,000 tonnes

The total US garlic crop is worth around $100 million every year

The town of Gilroy in California produces over 90% of the entire US garlic crop

It is said that over 70% of the UK population use garlic and that over 30% use it at least once a week

China, Thailand, Spain and Egypt produce the most garlic

Italian garlic is cultivated in the Po Valley region

The main producer in Britain is a farm on The Isle of Wight

People in the South of England eat twice-as-much garlic as those in Northern France!

Garlic is a prescription medicine in Germany, Holland and Denmark

The German Federal Health Board declares that garlic has "No known side effects" but if you eat too much you might stink!

Also in Germany garlic is a licensed medicine for "preventing age related deterioration of the circulation"

In Germany the Health Ministry has declared that garlic is a medicine for "assisting in the dietary treatment of raised blood fat levels"

German folk medicine has always said that eating large quantities of garlic can combat cancer

Garlic appears in the official drug guides in both Spain and Switzerland

The allicin content of Egyptian garlic is less than 0.03% but Egypt is one of the largest exporter's in the world

Chinese garlic can sometimes produce over 0.6% allicin

Spanish experts suggest that you get more total sulphur from garlic if it is organically grown

In China around the turn of the century it was traditional to eat two steamed meat patties called "chiao-tze" laden with garlic every day

In a study in Russia in 1972 garlic was used as an inhalant to treat over 200 cases of lung tuberculosis - successfully!

In India certain groups are forbidden to eat garlic and evidence shows that they have much higher cholesterol levels than those who do eat garlic regularly

Afro-Americans in the rural South have used garlic to prevent and treat high blood pressure since the days of slavery

In Russia garlic is officially recommended as a preventative against influenza

Researchers in America have shown that garlic can release 15 different kinds of antioxidant chemicals

A report in *Science Weekly* magazine in Frankfurt showed that freshly cut garlic could kill bacteria at a distance of 20cm by its vapour alone!

In the last week of July in the town of Gilroy in California the world's biggest garlic festival is held every year

In Poland evidence for the use of garlic for middle ear infections is documented

In Australia garlic was used recently to cure Ringworm infections and did so 3 times faster than modern drugs

In 1982 researchers in America showed that injected garlic extract could reduce the growth of liver cancers in animals by over 50%

Native Indians from America used garlic to treat bee stings and scorpion bites

In Spain it is traditional for bullfighter's to carry garlic in to the arena so as to prevent the bull from charging

The woods on parts of Dartmoor in England have large amounts of wild garlic growing in them and the aroma produced is very subtle and healthy!

In Italy garlic is eaten three times a day to relieve sore necks!

The wild precursor to the garlic we know today was called Allium longicuspis and was found growing in narrow gorges to the west of Samarkand

When Chinese garlic (rich in allicin) is grown in other parts of the world it loses its ability to produce lots of allicin

Dr Albert Schwietzer used garlic to treat cholera and typhoid in Africa

In America garlic has its own newsletter "The Garlic Press" as a guide to its propagation and continued consumption

In California there is a Society called "The Lovers of the Stinking Rose" where they have garlic in every course at their society luncheons

In Cairo street sellers call out "*Infa e' thoum*" - garlic is useful

In India garlic is worn to fight off evil spirits

Some general facts and figures

It is believed that around 500 species of allium still exist today. Once there were over 1000 species of onion, leeks, shallots chives and garlic

Garlic has been shown to be effective in the treatment of lead, mercury, cadmium, and arsenic poisoning

Garlic is known as "The Stinking Rose" because of all the smelly sulphur compounds it can produce

Garlic is the richest source of organically bound selenium, which has been shown to provide some protection against heavy-metal poisoning

Hang up garlic around the home to help get rid of bad smells!

A number of successful case studies on Tuberculosis were published in a book entitled *The Treatment of Tuberculosis with Oleum Allii* written by Dr William Minchin

Garlic has also been used to treat cases of Cryptococcal meningitis, a disease which is often fatal and without any side effects

When you cut an onion a compound called propenyl sulphenic acid makes you cry; there is much less of it in garlic but it is there nonetheless

Researchers have found that garlic oil is less effective than raw or powdered garlic at treating infections

Many people have reported directly that taking garlic, in any form, keeps colds away - over years and years!

There have been studies where up to 70 cloves of garlic were ingested in a day with no sign of any side effects!

Garlic is an elixir against the three humours of Indian Medicine: wind, phlegm and bile

Common or local names for garlic include – Poor Man's Treacle, Devils Posy, Witch Poison, Camphor of the Poor and the Food of Love

To prevent a vampire from leaving his grave at night, place a bulb of garlic in his mouth!

Garlic is also known as ramsons or buckrams because its smell is as strong as a ram

Try rubbing a cut clove of garlic on the edges of broken china plates, apply medium pressure and they will stick together!

For medical research the *British Medical Journal* says that carefully dried sliced cloves retain their potency, but extracts or oils prepared by using steam distillation may have little activity

As a cure for nightmares mince a clove or two of garlic into a bottle of red wine and take a glass each evening

The director of the National Cancer Institute in America has said that garlic has the most potential of all foods as a cancer fighting substance

Tibetan monks are forbidden to stay in the monastery if they eat garlic!

A recipe for marital fidelity - both eat garlic!

Historical facts

When Mount Vesuvius erupted and buried Pompeii the surviving Romans found garlic bulbs preserved in the ashes!

In the First World War the British Government offered one shilling per pound of garlic grown as it was used to prevent wounds turning septic

During both World Wars garlic was used to treat typhus and dysentery

In World War I physicians made their own ground garlic powder tablets as a cure for dysentery - this avoided the burning sensation found in the mouth when soldiers were told to eat raw garlic

When garlic was used for treating dysentery it was often mixed with some cold yoghurt or sour cream

Garlic was used by the invading armies from France in 1066 for adding strength and stamina to the archers

Thomas Culpepper the famous physician described garlic as 'the herb all heal' in 1642

Several bulbs of garlic were found in King Tutankhamen's tomb when it was opened – presumably to ward off evil spirits

Slaves building the pyramids went on strike when daily rations of garlic were stopped

During a flu epidemic in 1965 in Russia the Moscow Evening News told everyone to "eat more garlic"

In the 2nd century BC the Chinese called garlic the barbarian or Hu da suan

The renowned Egyptologist Sir William Petrie was able to trace garlic back to 3750 BC well before the Pharaohs arrived in Egypt

The first chemistry experiments on garlic were performed in 1844 by a Professor Wertheim when an "evil smelling oil" was produced after passing steam through a bubbling garlic mush

I have been spending some weeks of dissipation in London, and was transformed by Circe's cup not into a brute but into a beau. I am now eating the herb moly (garlic) in the country - Sidney Smith, 1813

Shakespeare called garlic the food of rustics (Henry IV Part I, III, I and A Winter's Tale IV, 3)

"Our apothecary's shop is our garden full of pot-herbs, and our doctor is a clove of garlic," an anonymous author wrote in 1615.

The sixteenth century herbalist William Turner recorded garlic as growing "in woddes about Bath"

According to legend the Romans liked to plant sweet violet (also known as love-in-idleness) next to garlic and onions

Shakespeare wrote in A Midsummer Night's Dream that actors should 'eat no onions nor garlic, for we are to utter sweat breath'

Garlic was mentioned in 22 Herbal remedies in the Codex Ebers, an Egyptian medical papyrus of 1550 BC

In early Roman times the sweet odour of garlic was associated with labourers and the lower classes

The 17th Century herbalist, Parkinson, advocated Garlic as an antidote to drinking poison such as hemlock or wolfs bane

In 1875 the distinguished botanist, Eduard von Regel, published an account of over 250 species belonging to the Allium group

In India the oldest Sanskrit manuscript tells the story of the origins of garlic (AD 350-375)

Henry IV of France (1566 – 1593) chewed Garlic consistently and was said to have had "a breath that could fell an ox at 20 paces"

The introduction of the famous Bower manuscript deals exclusively with garlic and dates back to the sixth century BC

In Tibet the Caravan men used garlic as an antidote to altitude sickness

The Roman poet Horace wrote a hymn of hate against garlic

Garlic originated in Siberia in the Kirgiz desert

Garlic has been established as a medicine for thousands of years and was well recognised by the Egyptians, Babylonians, Greeks, Chinese, Vikings, Indians and Romans.

In India, Rahu, King of the Asuras stole the elixir of life and the God Vishnu cut off his head. It is told that Rahu drank the elixir and his throat stayed with his severed head - and from the blood that was spilt sprang garlic!

Mohammed says that when Satan went from the Garden of Eden, garlic appeared from the ground where his left foot rested and onion at his right

During the plague in Marseilles in 1722 thieves who robbed the dead maintained that eating garlic protected them from infection. Hence "Four Thieves' Vinegar" was invented

Lepers acquired the name "pilgarlic" as they were made to peel cloves for their own consumption

Pliny, the ancient Greek physician, names 61 ailments that could be treated with garlic

In the Middle East garlic was carried as a talisman. In Chinese mythology, garlic is a ruse against the Evil Eye!

Garlic was used to treat rabies in the 16th and 17th century

In 1933 in Eastern Europe, researchers found that garlic could not only stop atherosclerosis in cats but could also reverse it

The First World Congress on the health significance of garlic was held in Washington DC in 1990

At the turn of the century garlic was also used in Ireland to treat tuberculosis

The Greek writer Aristophanes wrote plays containing jokes about garlic including its medical uses

Pliny claimed that taking pounded garlic with coriander and neat wine was a powerful Roman aphrodisiac!

In Anglo-Saxon day's flag and feverfew, garlic and radish were all used to help bronchial conditions

In Siberia the locals used to pay their taxes in garlic bulbs

Chocolate covered garlic was served at The White House by Eleanor Roosevelt

Louis Pasteur noted that garlic juice had an antimicrobial effect many years before Alexander Fleming invented penicillin.

During the reign of Ramses III, in Egypt, garlic was used to preserve bodies!

The Bower manuscript also says that: when women can no longer wear the cool seductive clothes of summer and rooftop parties are too cold then and only then should the Festival of Garlic be held

When the Roman's first brought garlic to England it was used as a flavouring for goose

Following a visit to France the poet Shelley wrote, "What do you think? Young women of rank eat - you will never guess what - garlick!

In Ancient Greece garlic was used as a diuretic and as a cleanser of the digestive system

The 2nd century Greek physician Galen described garlic as "theriacum rusticorum" or "poor man's treacle"

Professor Wesselin Petkov from Bulgaria was the first person to study the effect of garlic on blood circulation when in 1949 he added it to rabbits that had developed blocked arteries.

Since 1948 over 1500 scientific papers on garlic have been published

The First International Symposium on garlic research was held in Luneberg in Germany in 1989

Garlic hints and tips for health

Check exactly how much garlic is contained in your supplement, as some are virtually 'garlic free'

Garlic is a harmless medicinal food taken by millions for thousands of years without any major problems

Garlic products should not be given to children under six years old, but of course garlic may be added to their diet

Take your garlic supplements with meals to reduce the risk of developing an odour

Garlic is a cardio-protective as it can thin the blood, reduce blood pressure and cholesterol

Garlic can reduce levels of harmful cholesterol (LDL-Cholesterol) in your body

Generally the higher your cholesterol the more likely garlic is to reduce it

The well-known journal *Annals of Medicine* suggests that as little as half a clove a day may be enough to reduce cholesterol

In Japan garlic preparations are accepted as a means of reducing blood pressure

Garlic is as good as aspirin at thinning the blood but unlike aspirin it won't rot your stomach

Garlic can prevent the build up of fat in your coronary arteries

It is estimated that the incidence of stroke in the UK could be reduced by 30-40% if allicin producing garlic supplements were used by everyone at risk

Taken regularly garlic can help your circulation by thinning the blood and making it less likely to clot

Studies confirm that garlic can reduce blood pressure (both systolic and diastolic) by up to 10%

Garlic contains adenosine, which acts on the blood protein fibrin, which makes blood clot

Adding garlic extracts to human blood cells that are heavily diseased with atheroma will reduce the fat content substantially and return the cells to normal

In some countries (like Spain and France) the population regularly consumes garlic every day in almost every meal – their coronary heart disease rate is much lower than the UK or USA

Ingestion of garlic leads to immediate and large reductions in blood clotting

According to Dr D Kritchevsky at the Wistar Institute in Philadelphia garlic slows down the manufacture of cholesterol and other fats in the liver

Garlic is also able to break up blood clots very quickly, particularly in people who have already had a heart attack

Garlic is an excellent anti-blood clotting agent as it can thin the blood and make it less likely to stick together

Although garlic thins the blood experiments have shown that taking large quantities will not cause excessive bleeding

Experiments in Oxford showed that eating garlic quickly stopped patients blood platelets from sticking together

Garlic has been used much like smelling salts - to revive ladies who faint!

Garlic can reduce the number of harmful free radicals circulating in your body

Garlic is a potent anti-bacterial and can kill some of the most resistant and harmful bacteria known to man

As far as we know no organism has ever developed a resistance to garlic

The most garlic-sensitive bacteria is the frightening *Bacillus anthracis*; which produces the deadly poison anthrax

Garlic is as effective as Chloramphenicol (a powerful antibiotic) and can even kill strains that are resistant to it

Studies have shown that garlic can kill deadly human parasites including *Entamoeba histolytica* and *Giardia lamblia*

Garlic has been shown to be as effective as the common antibiotic Metronidazole which is use to treat amoebic dysentery - garlic is of course much cheaper and easier to produce!

Take garlic capsules to help ward off mosquitoes

Rub garlic paste over an aching tooth and it will remove the pain

Continued handling of garlic can cause skin rashes

Garlic is a known carminative as it stimulates the secretion of digestive juices and is known to remove "the wind"

Garlic can protect your blood cells against damage from various pollutants such as lead, mercury, copper and aluminium

Garlic is an expectorant and can therefore be used for treating asthma, bronchitis and catarrh

Put a clove of garlic in a child's shoe to prevent whooping cough (the smell will be excreted through the lungs!)

Garlic has also proved beneficial to asthma sufferers by opening up the airways

Garlic will prevent tummy bugs and rid the dreaded diarrhoea

As a cure for constipation try eating a clove of garlic every day

In patients who have developed AIDS, one complication is resistant diarrhoea. Taking garlic tablets stops this problem completely according to researchers at Guy's Hospital in London

Researchers in America have shown that garlic can stimulate the number of natural killer cells in our bodies.

Garlic can significantly increase the number of important T cells that AIDS patients lack

Some physicians advocate using garlic to inhibit human *cytomegalovirus*, which attacks people with poorly developed immune systems

People who are regular garlic consumers tend to have more white blood cells and are able to fight infections more easily

Taking a large dose of garlic capsules will prevent a cold coming on and will stop it completely

When you feel a cold coming on either take a large dose of your garlic supplement or cut a clove and sniff the garlic for a few minutes

For mouth ulcers chop the end off a clove of garlic, dip it into a pot of natural yoghurt and apply it directly to the mouth ulcer – it will sting but only for a moment!

Italian voice coaches recommend raw garlic as a throat tonic to make the voice stronger

For hemorrhoids scrape a clove to produce juice, insert it into the rectum and leave overnight!

Garlic is the only antibiotic which at the same time as killing bacteria also encourages digestion and protects the body against poisons produced by the infection

If you have Athlete's foot then simply crush some garlic cloves into a piece of lint and apply regularly to the affected area

Soak your fingernails in warm water containing a cut clove of garlic. It will keep them strong and prevent splitting

Some people are allergic to garlic in any form - even the minute amounts used in some salad dressings

In America, the National Cancer Institute has developed a $20 million programme to study the effects of various plants including garlic

Components of garlic can stop cancer-causing agents from binding on to human breast cells

Cancer studies have shown that the more garlic you eat the lower your risk of developing various stomach cancers

Compounds of garlic are used in Cancer patients to reduce the carcinogenic effect of prescription medicines

Recent results indicate that garlic may be able to help fight bladder cancer by inhibiting the growth of cancer cells

Investigations have shown that some of the components of garlic can mitigate the effects of some of the most potent carcinogens known including those found in cigarette smoke

The skin cancer cells found in Burkett's Lymphoma are reported to be susceptible to garlic

Investigations have shown that garlic can reduce blood sugar levels

Garlic is good for diabetes as it will help normalise the level of blood fats that can get out of control

Garlic has been shown to be almost 60% as effective as the diabetic drug Tolbutamide

Garlic is an excellent anti-oxidant that can reduce harmful free radicals circulating in your body

Garlic is the only antibiotic, which at the same time as killing bacteria also encourages digestion and protects the body against poisons produced by the infection

Garlic can kill the bacteria responsible for skin, lung, throat and mouth infections

Garlic can be used to calm bites and stings – just crush 3 cloves of garlic and mix with some warm water. Dab it onto the affected parts

Mix garlic with lard and apply to your skin to help pimples and boils disappear

Try rubbing corns with a cut clove of garlic every day until the corn disappears

Rub some garlic juice on to finger warts and they will disappear

If you have a verruca, try cutting a thin slice from a garlic clove and place it over the verruca - continue this for a week and the verruca will disappear

Garlic has been shown to increase blood flow to the nail fold capillaries

Improved circulation to the arteries in the eye has also been demonstrated with garlic

If you have problems with poor circulation take garlic every day to improve the situation

Garlic has been proven to help patients with intermittent claudication (lack of blood reaching the limbs) to walk further!

Garlic will start to work immediately but you need to persevere for several months before you see real benefits to your circulation

Garlic can improve blood circulation to the skin by as much as 47%

Remember it's the smelly part of garlic that is the most active - allicin

Amazingly even the blood of people who eat a lot of garlic can kill bacteria!

A cure for earache   soak a peeled clove of garlic in olive oil for a few minutes and place it in your ear. The ache will vanish!

Garlic cough mixture   crush one clove of garlic into some honey or syrup. Take one tablespoon twice a day

In Russia they place a whole head of garlic (all the cloves) in a cup of milk to treat whooping cough

Chew a clove alone every day to help sinus infections

Gargle with crushed cloves of garlic mixed with brewed sage and warm water – an excellent remedy for tonsillitis or excessive mucous

In Poland garlic has been shown to be effective against recurrent catarrh and chronic bronchitis

Use garlic as an inhalant for nasal congestion. Take three or four cloves, crush them and add a little apple vinegar. Then pour on a pint of boiling water and inhale the fumes

Raw garlic is often useful for treating acne and eczema as it tends to remove the internal impurities that cause the problem

Garlic does not interact with other prescription medicines

Chew raw garlic every day to build up your strength

When new Mother's eat lots of garlic their new-born babies breast feed for longer

In Israel garlic is given to women for 10 days after childbirth to prevent infections and to help the uterus return to normal

In Eastern Europe it is traditional for women to put garlic on their pillows during childbirth and in their children's clothes at baptism

Garlic juice and wild thyme can be used as a prophylactic against snake bites

Take garlic tablets or capsules on holiday to ward off mosquitoes

Scorpion bites produce harmful enzymes so they can be treated by cutting a clove of garlic and spreading it onto the wound

Garlic can rid the body of ringworm and pinworm although it is rarely used to treat this common Third World condition

Prolonged contact with fresh garlic, particularly on the gums or on wounds, can cause blistering. However sometimes it is used this way deliberately to draw out poisons - hence its use as a rubefacient

To help rheumatism, try rubbing a peeled clove of garlic over the affected joint

Garlic components

One clove of garlic can produce a head (or bulb) containing up to around 20 cloves

Three pounds of fresh garlic will yield one pound of dried garlic

Raw garlic contains water, fat, sugars, pectin, cellulose, mucilage, total ash, acid soluble ash, peptides and proteins

Garlic contains minerals such as selenium, sodium, potassium, iron, cobalt, zinc, nitrogen, calcium, chromium, sulphur, magnesium, phosphorus copper and iodine

The vitamins A, B_1, B_2 and C plus zinc and selenium are present in Garlic thus accounting for its antioxidant properties

One clove of garlic contains between 1 and 4 calories!

Garlic is approximately 60% water

Garlic contains at least 9 parts per million of Selenium

Garlic contains around 10 different sugars including glucose, fructose and arabinose

Garlic in storage and cooking

The great chef, Marcel Boulestin maintained that peace and happiness begin where garlic is used in cooking

Appearances can be deceptive since small cloves of garlic often produce the most flavour!

Chef's believe that you get different aromas from garlic depending upon how you crush it

Garlic bulbs are best kept by hanging up by its stalk in a cool dry airy dark cupboard

Please don't store garlic in the refrigerator as it deadens the flavour

A garlic press adds a crude metallic taste to crushed garlic and is best avoided

Add garlic to your weekly roasts for extra flavour

Rub a crushed clove around your salad bowl to add that extra flavour without overpowering your meal

Raw garlic's potency can vary by as much as 13 fold, so pick a strong well cultivated garlic – Spanish garlic is currently the best

In Spain fresh garlic shoots are a delicacy fried for tapas

Buy garlic heads that are plump and unbruised as they will give the best flavour

Reject any bulbs that have started to dry out as they will have lost their flavour

Garlic can be bought as flakes, pieces, powder and pickled

Bury three peeled and pressed cloves in half a cup of sea salt. Leave it for a few days in a screw top jar. Remove the garlic and use the salt as a seasoning

Add peeled cloves to a jar of oil refrigerate and leave for 2-3 days before using. Brush on foods before they are grilled or sautéed

Add peeled cloves of garlic to white wine vinegar and keep for 2-3 days before using in salad dressings

Dehydrated garlic is virtually odourless but when water is added the flavour returns almost completely

When boiling vegetables add several whole cloves of garlic into the water to add a subtle aroma

Garlic is often used as a preservative for cooked meats and for summer picked fruits

Don't burn your garlic as it will smell awful – it singes much more quickly than Onions

Boiling garlic almost completely removes the odour

Fresh garlic will irritate the stomach so try taking it with a little water

When cooking with garlic in Spain it is common practice to squash the cloves under a knife before chopping and so produce a slightly different flavour

When you chew raw garlic take a little water with it to lessen the burning taste

Garlic can upset some people's digestion so beware particularly if you eat it raw

Chewing cardamom seeds can sometimes remove the garlic smell from your breath. Chew parsley after garlic or suck a peppermint to prevent the dreaded 'foul breath'

Another recorded breath freshener used after eating garlic is the bitter herb rue

Even though garlic has a powerful smell and taste it is virtually non-toxic

Another time worn remedy for avoiding garlic breath – chew aniseed

Hang garlic by the kitchen door to keep fairies away from the butter churn

Chicken soup laced with garlic is called "Jewish penicillin"

As an aphrodisiac garlic should be pounded with fresh coriander and taken in neat wine!

As you add more garlic to your diet the less any smell will be noticed

Try swallowing a clove of garlic before you have your garlic-flavoured meal and you will smell as sweet as anyone who eats no garlic!

When garlic leaves its characteristic odour on your hands wash them with lemon juice to remove it

The well known cook, Mrs Beeton, proclaimed in one of her books that "The smell of garlic is generally considered offensive"

In many parts of Southern Europe (particularly Italy) garlic is found in almost every dish!

The national food of Peru is said to be garlic eaten with bread and potatoes

Life without garlic is tasteless!

Garlic in the garden

Garlic is a member of the lily family and its English name is thought to come from the Anglo-Saxon "Gar-Leac" or Spear Plant

Garlic is also known as *Allium Sativum* and there are over 500 members of the *Alliaceae* or onion family

Garlic was first grown in English gardens in about 1540

Garlic can grow up to 3ft tall although wild garlic tends to be shorter

Plant your garlic cloves in November as they tend to produce bigger bulbs the following Spring

When growing your own garlic remember the plant prefers light sandy soil. If your soil is too rich the leaves will grow too much and your bulbs will be poor quality

When growing garlic, avoid soggy soil and over-watering

Make sure you plant your cloves pointed side up!

Garlic can easily be grown in pots and window boxes, provided that their is adequate drainage

When your plants have flowered remove the heads and when the tops begin to go brown its time to harvest!

Garlic cannot fertilise itself by pollination and rarely produces seed

Aqueous garlic extracts can be sprayed on to a variety of crops to act as a foliar and root feed

Plant your garlic near carrots or roses and you will protect them from blight. Alternatively, spray early with aqueous garlic extracts to prevent blight, black spot and moulds

Scatter pieces of garlic amongst grain and it will help to keep weevils away

Spray garlic juice onto your plants to keep downy mildew away

Aqueous garlic extracts contain plenty of beneficial sulphur that can unlock the full potential of plants and soil allowing maximum plant feeding efficiency

Protect your cucumbers from rust by feeding regularly with water that has had garlic soaking in it for several hours

The sixteenth century herbalist Tusser proclaimed "set garlicke and beans at St Edmund the King". St Edmund's day is November 15th so plant your garlic then!

As the plant grows, bend back or break off the main stem to increase the size of the bulb

Garlic can be caught by blackspot and clove rotting caused by the fungi *Fusarium*

Garlic plants can also be attacked by nematodes, mites and the garlic *mosaic* virus

Garlic grows well next to plums and cherries but avoid placing it near peas and beans

One of the easiest varieties of garlic to grow comes from Clermont-Ferrand in the Massif Central in France

If you need a supply of the finest English garlic seed contact Mersley-Boswell Farms in Newchurch Isle of Wight

Garlic bulbs are actually quite tender and will bruise easily so take care when you pull them out of the ground

Use sheep manure, which is rich in sulphur, to help your garlic grow strong and healthy!

To get rid of moles try placing peeled and cut cloves of garlic in their holes

Garlic for animals

Give garlic powder to your dogs and cats to prevent fleas and ticks

Feed garlic to horses to 'sweeten' their breath

Garlic is used in Ireland and France to strengthen racehorses and improve circulation

Pigeon racers add garlic to bird seed to add stamina and speed

Chickens lay bigger eggs if garlic is added to their feed - be sure to stop adding garlic as the hens begin to lay otherwise your eggs will be garlic flavoured!

Garlic feeding has been used in animals to minimise the amount of lead in the meat of food animals, which have been reared in lead polluted environment

In the USA both pigs and chickens are fed garlic to raise the levels of HDL (protective fats) in their blood

In rabbits given large amounts of cholesterol when fed with garlic their reduction in cholesterol was over 29%

Hungarian jockeys fastened cloves of garlic to the bits of their horses, believing that other horses would keep away (so eventually everyone did it!)

If crows eat garlic it stupefies them!

In France when a horse develops clots in the legs it is treated with a diet of garlic and onions

Add garlic capsules to your dogs dinner and it will help to get rid of worms – look for that product that contains 100% allicin yield

Farmers have found all around the world that garlic will help to keep their livestock free from ticks and other parasites

Garlic definitely repels vampire bats; in South America where these creatures live it is reported that they will not attack horses that are fed on garlic!

'The heart of Garlic' – Allicin

Allicin (garlic's main active ingredient) was first isolated in 1944 by the chemist Cavallito.

Garlic's principle active agent is allicin

Your body will get much more benefit if you can eat garlic that has been cut into slices as crushing will destroy much of the active 'allicin'

Independent research confirms that many garlic supplements cannot provide ANY of the garlic's active principal allicin

The most effective way to use garlic without the smell is to look for products that guarantee a 100% allicin yield

Conclusion...

In this book you have read how allicin, "Nature's Antibiotic", can kill TB, Smallpox, MRSA, *Streptococcus* species and many many more troubling microorganisms, with the additional benefit of strengthening your immune system to prevent further attack and yet not disrupting or destroying your existing healthy bacteria.

There's a great deal going on in terms of research and clinical trials. Barely do I finish a draft of this book when I immediately have to revise it as many studies on allicin, added to a wide range of other active raw ingredients, are underway.

Aside from this crucial requirement for a natural antibiotic/antifungal/antiviral, allicin therapy has begun to be evaluated for the prevention and treatment of the world's two biggest killer diseases: cancer and coronary heart disease.

In those nations where garlic consumption, both cooked and raw, is a strong part of the culture and daily life, much lower coronary death rates and significant protection from cancer is evident.

Obviously, there are many other factors involved, but this book, for the first time, considers the broader picture of medically approved studies and confirms what great physicians, herbalists and healers have suggested for thousands of years, namely, that something garlic produces is good for human health. Now at long last, after 80 years of trying to release the "mother substance" – the HEART of garlic – allicin is finally available in sufficient quantities to act as a natural body!

Bibliography...

Oxford Medical Dictionary Fourth Edition

Darbyshire B., Henry R.J., Differences in *fructan* content and synthesis in some *Allium* species, *New Phytol.* 87 (1981) 249-256.

Koch H.P., Lawson L.D., Garlic, the science and therapeutic application of *Allium sativum* L. and related species, in: Retford D.C. (Ed.),

Williams and Wilkins, Baltimore, 1996, pp. 1-233.

Cavallito C., Bailey J.H., Allicin, the antibacterial principle of *Allium sativum*.

Isolation, physical properties and antibacterial action, J. Am. Chem. Soc. 66 (1944) 1944-1952.

Block E., The chemistry of garlic and onion, Sc. Am. 252 (1985) 94-99.

Stoll A., Seebeck E., Chemical investigations of alliin, and the specific principle of garlic, *Adv. Enzymol.* 11 (1951) 377-400.

Ellmore G.S., Feldberg R.S., Alliin lyase localisation in bundle sheaths of garlic clove (*Allium sativum*), *Am. J. Bat.* 81(1994) 89-94.

Rabinkov A., Xiao-Zhu Z., Grafl G., Galili G., Mirelman D., Alum lyase (alliinase) from garlic (*Allium sativum*):Biochemical characterisation and cDNAcloning, *Appl.Biochem.Biotechnol.* 48 (1994) 149-171.

Van Damme 5.3.24., Smeets K., Torrekens S., Van Leaven F., Peumans W.J., Isolation and characterisation of alliinase cDNA clones from garlic (*Alliumsativum* L.) and related species, *Eur.J. Biochem.* 209 (1992) 751-757.

Rabinkov A., Wilchek M., Mirelman D., Alumnae (alum lyase) from garlic (*Allium sativum*) is glycosylated at ASN146 and forms a complex with a garlic mannosespecific lectin, *Glyco conj.* 3. 12 (1995) 690-698.

Uchida Y., Takahashi T., Sato N., The characteristics of the antibacterial activity of garlic, *Jpn J. Antibiotics* 28 (1975) 638-642.

Celiini L, Di Campli B., Masulli M., Di Bartolomeo S., Aliocati N., Inhibition of *Helicobacter pylori* by garlic extract (*Allium sativum*), FEMS Immenol. Med. Micrbiol 13 (1996) 273-277

Gonzalez-Fandos F., Garcia-Lopez Mi.., Sierra Mi., Otero A., Staphylococcal growth and enterotoxins (A-D) and thermonuclease synthesis in the presence of dehydrated garlic,J. *Appl. Bacteriol.* 77 (1994) 549-552.

Girnenez MA., Solanes RE., Girneriez D.F., Growth of *Clostridium botulinum* in media with garlic, *Rev. Argent. Microbioi.* 20 (1988) 17-24.

Holzgartner H, Schmidt U, Kuhn U Congress Abstract *Eur Jnl Clin Res* 3A 1992:8

Brosche T and Platt D (1991) Garlic *BMJ*; 303; 785

Rabinkov A.,. Miron T., Konsrantinovski L., Wilchek M., Mirelman D., Weiner L., The mode of action of allicin: trapping of radicals and interaction with thiol containing proteins, *Biochim. Biophys. Acts* 1379 (1998) 233-244.

Abdullah TH, Kirkpatrick DH, Carter J; Enhancement of Natural Killer Cell activity in AIDS patients; *D Z Onkologie* 21;52-53

Josling P *Advances in Natural Therapy* (2001) 18; 189-193

Steinmetz et al., (1994) Vegetable fruit and colon cancer in The IOWA Women's Health Study. *Am. J. Epidemiol.* 139: 1-15.

Eccles R. Common Cold Centre Cardiff.

Koch and Lawson in *Garlic – The Science and Therapeutic Application of Allium Sativum L and Related Species.* Williams & Wilkins; 1996.

Ankri & Mirelman. *Microbes Infect.* 1999;2:125-129.

Hanley & Fenwick. *J Plant Foods.* 1985;6:211-238.

Data on file. Garlic Centre, East Sussex, UK.

Acknowledgement

I should like to record my grateful thanks to Dr Ron Cutler from The University of East London for the many contributions he has made to the writing of this book.

Index...

a

Other titles available from the same author

Special Report on the world's first Pre and Probiotic combination for digestive health. Designed to restore a natural balance to your digestive system. This 30 page special report will be required reading for anyone with IBS, diverticulitis, food intolerances or other general digestive disorders.

Special Report on the incidence, cause and the use of allicin powder for the treatment of Candida infection. 30 pages.

Special report on the antiparasitic properties of allicin. Activity can be expected against a wide range of parasite infestations including Lyme, head lice, Giardia, mosquitoes and liver flukes. 40 pages.

Special report on cancer, very detailed on the possible causes (including viral) treatment options and how allicin powder and ellagic acid may help as a cancer preventative. 40 pages.

100% Allicin yield brands sold around the world

Country	Brand names for 100% Allicin yield products
Belgium	Allimax
Canada	Allimax
Denmark	Garcin
Holland	Knoflox-Allimax
Hong Kong	Alliforce
Japan	Alliforce
Norway	Weissin
UK & Ireland	Alliforce & Allimax
USA	Allimax, Alli-C, AlliPRO, LifeSpice, Detoxal[21]

Useful Information on garlic and allicin...

Sources for more information include:

The Garlic Centre
PO Box 29
Battle
East Sussex TN33 9BR
United Kingdom

Tel: 01424 892440
Email: garlic@mistral.co.uk

For additional information on allicin and 100% allicin products look at www.alliforce.com

ISBN 0-9546507-0-0 Barcode – 9 780954 650704